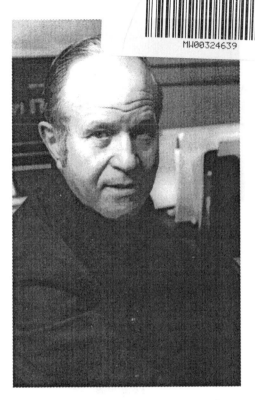

Sheldon Zerden, an account executive,
is the author of several books on
financial topics, including Best Books
on the Stock Market (winner of the
Book of the Year in Finance award
from the American Library Association
in 1973), Margin Power (1981) and The
Best of Health. He has combined the
analytical insight and thoroughness of a
stock market strategist with a serious
interest in health issues and more than
ten years of research to produce a work
of lasting importance.

The Cholesterol Hoax

101+ Lies
by
Sheldon Zerden

Library of Congress Cataloging-in-Publication Data

Zerden, Sheldon
      The Cholesterol Hoax: 101+ LIes / Sheldon Zerden.
            p.   cm.
      Includes bibliographical references.
      ISBN 0-9640104-2-9 (alk. paper)
      1. Coronary heart disease--Etiology. 2. Cholesterol -
      - Physiciological effect.   3. Cholesterol--Pathophysiology.   I. Title
RC685.C6Z47   1997   97-40599
616.1' 23071--dc21   CIP

Cover Designer: Alane Kitchen
In-House Editors
Typesetters: A M Business Services

Published by
BRIDGER HOUSE PUBLISHERS, INC.
P.O. Box 2208, Carson City, NV 89702, 1-800-729-4131

Printed in the United States of America
10 9 8 7 6 5 4 3 2 1

ACKNOWLEDGEMENTS

The text of this book would not be possible without the work of a great many people. I have been inspired by the integrity and dedication of researchers and scientists whose lives have enriched us all. During the years I worked on "The Best of Health", I received the support of two Nobel Laureates, Linus Pauling and Albert Szent-Gyorgyi. Dr. Abram Hoffer, Dr. Carl C. Pfeiffer, Dr. Robert C. Atkins, Dr. John Yudkin and Roger Williams. All were helpful. The list reads like a hall of fame in the nutrition field.

The cholesterol paradigm intrigued me and I couldn't understand how there could be such a strong consensus. I then found that there were people of substance who dissented. I read all I could about the controversy. The result was this work which should alert the public to the truth.

Many of the facts revealed here are culled from the great array of books in the bibliography. I owe a great debt of gratitude to Dr. George V. Mann for his life of dedication to science and his "Coronary Heart Disease: The Dietary Sense and Nonsense." I also learned a lot from Thomas J. Moore's "The Cholesterol Myth." Dr. Edward R. Pinckney and Cathey Pinckney put the spotlight on hydrogenated vegetable oils in "The Cholesterol Controversy." The most thorough treatment on the cholesterol deception is Russell L. Smith's "The Cholesterol Conspiracy." I would like to thank Joyce R. Green for her help.

I can't forget the years of continuing help of Fred A. Kummerow, Ph.D. and David Kritchevsky who offered support in the development of this work. And finally, I must offer thanks to my long suffering wife who was the sounding board for all my banter about cholesterol.

Sheldon Zerden
New York   1997

Dedication

To Daniel, Benjamin and Sarah

IMPASSE

Cholesterol is poisonous
so never, never eat it.
Sugar too, may murder you
there is no way to beat it.
And fatty food may do you in-
be certain to avoid it.
Some food was rich in vitamins
but processing destroyed it.

So let your life be ordered
by each documented fact
and die of malnutrition
but with arteries intact!

David Kritchevsky

TABLE OF CONTENTS

PREFACE

The diet-heart-cholesterol dogma is a fiction. It has grown and taken root in the consciousness of the American people with the nourishment of those forces in the scientific world, fundraising enterprises, government agencies, academia, industry and others. They have placed profit above truth, and pride above integrity.

George V. Mann M.D., who was an associate director of the Framingham study for three years, and recently retired from Vanderbilt University, characterized the cholesterol paradigm as follows:

> "Saturated fat and cholesterol in the diet are not the cause of coronary heart disease. That myth is the greatest deception of this century, perhaps of any century."

Heart disease is the number one killer in the United States accounting for 500,000 deaths. As many as 5 million coronary artery bypass procedures have been performed since 1970 at a total cost of $250 billion. In addition, there are 300,000 to 400,000 coronary angioplasty procedures every year at a cost of $10 billion to $20 billion. These procedures simply alleviate the symptoms of atherosclerosis, without curing the underlying disease.

The diet-heart-cholesterol hypothesis continues unabated with a $1,000,000,000 dollars a year in business. It is an industry that has led sane men of science astray and compromised the lives of almost everyone. For the American Heart Association, there is no turning back. If they do, the whole foundation of the diet-cholesterol consensus will go down in flames and take the massive food and pharmaceutical industries with them.

The present dilemma is a difficult one. Men of science

have abandoned the truth and joined the forces of greed. The giant cholesterol industry will make the task of honest men as difficult as scaling Mount Everest. The truth matters. It does to millions of Americans who deserve to know why it has been denied them for the last forty years. Our hope is that character and integrity will triumph over those who have deemed their own greed more important than the health of the American people.

LIE # 1

If you lower or eliminate cholesterol in your diet, your blood cholesterol will be lower.

FALSE

ANSWER: For the overwhelming majority of people, dietary cholesterol does not affect your blood (serum) cholesterol.

LIE # 2

The increase in coronary heart disease in the 20th century was caused by a growing consumption of cholesterol in the American diet.

FALSE

ANSWER: Americans have consumed approximately 600 mg. of cholesterol per day since 1909. The increasing heart attack rate cannot logically be blamed on dietary cholesterol.

LIE # 3

The more cholesterol you consume, the greater the risk of coronary heart disease.

FALSE

ANSWER: Rural Romanians have 10 to 20 times less coronary heart disease than Americans and they consume approximately 900 mg. of cholesterol per day, which is 300 mg more cholesterol than Americans. This indicates that there must be other factors than cholesterol in the diet of

Americans that increase the blood (serum) cholesterol level and the rate of coronary heart disease.

LIE # 4

Eggs increase your cholesterol.

FALSE

ANSWER: Three recent independent studies have shown that including two whole eggs per day in the diet had no significant effect on the serum cholesterol value of normal human subjects.

New York Times Article on September 24, 1977 by Gina Kolata "Scientists Ease up on Fear of Eggs." Two studies by Dr. Henry N. Ginsberg et al at Columbia University's College of Physicians and Surgeons found that young men and women who ate as many as three to four eggs a day for weeks on end had virtually no change in their blood cholesterol levels."*

*Ginsberg, Henry N. et al "A Dose-Response study of the effects of dietary cholesterol on fasting and postprandial lipid and post prandial lipid and lipoprotein metabolism in healthy young men." Arteriosclerosis Thromb. 1994: 14: 576-586.

Kummerow, F.A. et al "The influence of egg consumption on the serum cholesterol level in human subjects." American Journal of Clinical Nutrition 30:664, 1977.

Slater, G.J. et al "Plasma cholesterol and triglycerides in men with added eggs in the diet." Nutr. Rep. Int'l 14:249, 1976.

Porter, M.W. et al "Effect of dietary egg on serum cholesterol and Triglycerides of human males." American

Journal of Clinical Nutrition 30:490, 1977.

LIE # 5

If you want to lower your cholesterol, use margarine instead of butter.

FALSE

ANSWER: When margarine was tested against butter under clinically controlled conditions, the difference in serum cholesterol values was insignificant.*

    *Promise margarine clinical studies. Lever Brothers Co. 1972. Personal communications with Fred Kummerow at the Burnsides Research Laboratory, University of Illinois, Urbana-Champaign, Illinois.

LIE # 6

If you lower your cholesterol level, you will lengthen your life.

FALSE

ANSWER: There is no evidence at all that lowering your cholesterol will increase your longevity.

LIE # 7

High blood-cholesterol levels generally increase the risk of coronary heart disease among women.

FALSE

ANSWER: "For women, there was no relationship except in the middle decade of life (ages forty to fifty)."*

    *Thomas Dawber-First Study Director of the Framingham Heart Study.

LIE # 8

Cholesterol levels are most important in men and women over the age of fifty.

FALSE

ANSWER: The link between high blood-cholesterol levels and the increased risk of coronary heart disease weakened at age fifty and then disappeared entirely. Thus among the elderly, the group in whom most deaths from coronary heart disease occur, high cholesterol levels did not appear to be a risk factor.

    *Dawber, Thomas et al "Diet and the Regulation of Serum Cholesterol." Framingham Heart Study 1970

LIE # 9

Saturated fats increase blood cholesterol.

FALSE

ANSWER: According to a study titled, "Diet and the Regulation of Serum Cholesterol" Framingham researchers in 1970 concluded that the intake of saturated fats and overall calories had no effect on blood cholesterol. The study was never published in a scientific journal.

LIE # 10

Physical activity lowers blood cholesterol.

FALSE

ANSWER: Framingham researchers found that exercise made no difference. In fact, they found, "There is, in short, no suggestion of any relation between diet and the subsequent development of coronary heart disease in the study group."

LIE # 11

Coronary heart disease is caused by a high-fat, high cholesterol diet.

FALSE

ANSWER: Overwhelming evidence indicates that diet has little or nothing to do with coronary heart disease.

LIE # 12

The great epidemic of coronary heart disease during the first sixty years of this century was caused by increasing blood cholesterol levels. This increase was caused by our increased consumption of saturated fats and dietary cholesterol.

FALSE

ANSWER: This claim is not true and it cannot be supported by the facts. The basic fault with this thesis is that from 1900-1965, the cholesterol level of Americans was constant (about 220 mg/dl).

Kahn, Harold (National Heart and Lung Institute) Bethesda, MD American Journal of Clinical Nutrition, July 1970.

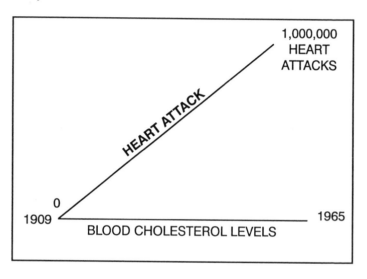

Study by Harold Kahn of the *National Heart and Lung Institute-Bethesda, MD* Reported in July 1970 *American Journal of Clinical Nutrition*

LIE # 13

If a person meticulously follows a low-fat, low-cholesterol diet all his life, and has normal blood pressure and avoids smoking, he can extend his life substantially.

FALSE

ANSWER: Dr. William Taylor et al obtained data from the Framingham Study which has followed and evaluated the community for fifty years. Researchers concluded that a lifelong cholesterol-lowering diet would extend life for a few weeks for young people with an initial cholesterol level of 180 mg/dl. If they had initial levels of over 300 mg/dl (5% of the population), they could expect a life extension of several months. This precludes an increase in deaths from other causes.

LIE # 14

Cholesterol-lowering diets increase your longevity.

FALSE

ANSWER: One editorial compared cholesterol-lowering diets to "rearranging the deck chairs on the Titanic."
M.H. Becker- "The Cholesterol Saga". Annals of Internal Medicine, 1987.

LIE # 15

Cholesterol is something to be feared.

FALSE

ANSWER: Cholesterol is absolutely essential to good health and is located in every cell in the body. The body contains about five ounces of cholesterol and only seven percent (one-third of an ounce) circulates in the blood.

Brown and Goldstein-New England Journal of Medicine, 1981.

LIE # 16

Diet is truly the cause of coronary heart disease.

FALSE

ANSWER: If diet is truly the cause of coronary heart disease, why is it necessary to conduct thousands of animal experiments and take eighty years to prove it? The answer has several parts. 1. Rabbits and other animals do not metabolize cholesterol like humans. Rabbits are vegetarian. 2. Rats and dogs, which metabolize cholesterol like humans, do not develop atherosclerosis when fed large amounts of cholesterol. 3. It was discovered that protein, carbohydrates and saturated and polyunsaturated fat can induce atherosclerotic disease. 4. In 1925, it was discovered that dietary cholesterol was not the principal source of blood cholesterol. Cholesterol was found to be manufactured in the body.

Ernst, N. And Levy, R.I. "Diet, Hyperlipidemia & Atherosclerosis." Modern Nutrition in Health & Disease. 6th ed. 1980.
5. A major difference in animals is that plaque is soft and disappears when the diet changes. Human plaque is hard and does not disappear when the diet changes.

Dr. Mark Altschule called the thousands of animal experiments "worthless". Dr. Myron Weisfeldt, the president of the American Heart Association in 1989 stated, "You can't say that reducing dietary cholesterol will reduce atherosclerosis."

LIE # 17

In 1961, the American Heart Association announced dietary recommendations for all persons "at risk for coronary heart disease (smokers, high blood cholesterol and high blood pressure)". They were told to reduce their consumption of fats and cholesterol and substitute polyunsaturated fats for saturated fats. In 1964, the American Heart Association announced recommendations for all Americans. 1. 300 mg. of cholesterol a day. 2. Total fat should be 30-35 percent of all calories. Did the American Heart Association mention restricting polyunsaturated fat to only 10 percent of total calories?

FALSE

ANSWER: After 1961, polyunsaturated fats were found to cause cancer in laboratory animals. The American Heart Association gave no reason for its restriction of polyunsaturated fats to 10 percent of total calories. Jane Brody, Dr. Frederick Stare and Dr. Jean Mayer encouraged the public to increase their intake of polyunsaturated fats over the next 18 years.

LIE # 18

The Inter-Society Commission for Heart Disease Resources was created by congress. It was an arm of the American Heart Association and the National Heart, Lung and Blood Institute (directed by a former president of the American Heart Association). The commission published a document recommending "The Prudent Diet" for all Americans. Is this diet beneficial for children?

FALSE

ANSWER: The American Academy of Pediatrics dissented. It said that serious harm to brain and mental development would result. The nervous system is heavily dependent on cholesterol.

LIE # 19

In 1984, the media praised the results of a ten year trial which used a drug to reduce blood cholesterol in a group of men with exceptionally high levels, to reduce coronary heart disease deaths. The results of the trial confirmed the truth that diet and drugs can decrease mortality in men with high cholesterol levels.

FALSE

ANSWER: The results were criticized by the medical community because though there were fewer coronary disease deaths reported in the treated group, the total number of deaths were the same. The National Heart, Lung and Blood Institute stressed the coronary heart disease difference but did not mention the mortality figures. The media praised the trial and indicated that all doubt was eliminated about the diet-coronary heart disease link, although the trial involved a drug, not a diet, and in spite of the fact that the cholesterol-lowering did not increase life expectancy.

LIE # 20

Diet/heart trials have proved conclusively that a high saturated fat, high cholesterol diet causes coronary heart disease.

FALSE

ANSWER: There have been 33 trials of the diet-heart hypothesis in the last 30 years. The evidence clearly shows that this is not a sound hypothesis. We cling to this disproven theory because of "pride, profit, and prejudice. How can these people admit they have made such a dreadful error? How can the American Heart Association admit its error? Its fund-raising program would self destruct! How can the bureaucrats admit they have wasted hundreds of millions of research money? These people are entangled in their own web of deception."*

*Mann, George, V., "Coronary Heart Disease"- The Dietary Sense and Nonsense- An Evaluation by Scientists- The Veritas Society

LIE # 21

The Maasai in Kenya and Tanzania are a nomadic people who consume mainly milk and meat in large quantities. They suffer from atherosclerosis and coronary heart disease.

FALSE

ANSWER: Their cholesterol levels are below 170 mg/dl and autopsies show little evidence of atheroma or plaque in their coronary arteries. They do not have heart disease.

LIE # 22

During the years 1955-1965, Dr. Ancel Keys used the statistical data of the World Health Organization (WHO) and selected the data from seven national reports that showed a linear relationship between estimated fat intake of the populations and the reported deaths from coronary heart disease. This proved that dietary fats and cholesterol caused coronary heart disease.

FALSE

ANSWER: Keys omitted the data from 15 nations in the same study that did not fit his preconceived notion. Such selection is not scientific, and is, of course cheating.

LIE # 23

Atherosclerosis is a condition characterized by clogged arteries that is caused by a buildup of cholesterol-containing plaque which leads to a heart attack.

FALSE

ANSWER: Atherosclerosis is more than just a matter of lipid deposition. One can find large amounts of smooth muscle, elastic tissue and collagen in lesions with relatively little fat, while in other areas, the lipid content is more pronounced. Moreover, one does not need an elevated blood cholesterol to produce a lesion.

Stehbens, W.E. "Coronary Heart Disease" Page 34.

LIE # 24

Polyunsaturated fat lowers cholesterol and therefore prevents coronary heart disease.

FALSE

ANSWER: After reviewing the dietary factors observed in Israel, Dr. McMichael concluded that "polyunsaturated fat does not prevent coronary heart disease, and might even be suspected of contributing to its development." S.H. Blondheim reported that experience in Israel cast doubt on the assumption that "eating a low-fat diet with a high ratio of polyunsaturated to saturated fatty acids protects against coronary heart disease." The Israeli experience showed that as immigrants increased their intake of vegetable oil, their serum lipids were increased and coronary heart disease increased as well.

The Bedouins in Israel, who had been eating animal fat in the desert began eating vegetable fat as they moved into the towns, and then their problems with coronary heart disease began.

McMichael, J. "Fats and Atheroma: An Inquest."
British Medical Journal 1, 173-175 (1975).
Blondheim, S.H. "Polyunsaturation of the Diet and the Development of Ischemic Heart Disease."
Talk given at MacDonald College of McGill University, 5 October 1983.

LIE # 25

Margarine is effective in preventing coronary heart disease.

FALSE

ANSWER: The trans-fatty acids found in margarine have been shown to raise LDL cholesterol levels and lower HDL levels. The literature has hinted that trans-fatty acids might have a role in coronary heart disease. Leren* reported an "alarming" post World War 2 increase in coronary heart disease in Norway concurrent with an increased fat intake in which 65 grams daily of subsidized hard margarine was a major component. The Scandinavians exported their butter and lard after World War 2 and ate hydrogenated soybean and whale oil because it was cheaper. This may explain the very high frequency of coronary heart disease, especially in Finland.

*Leren, P. "Prevention of Coronary Heart Disease: Some Results from the Oslo Secondary and Primary Intervention Studies. Journal of the American College of Nutrition, 8, 407-10 (1989).

LIE # 26

Cholesterol levels in rabbits can be lowered by feeding them partially hydrogenated vegetable oils.

FALSE

ANSWER: Even rabbits have problems with trans-fatty acids. A study by Kritchevsky's Group* described the larger cholesterol-raising and atheroma-producing effect of feeding rabbits partially hydrogenated soybean oil, especially when combined with animal protein. It should be noted that many of the animal studies that purport to show a saturated fat effect on cholesterol and atherogenesis have actually been feeding studies done with fats containing trans-fatty acids.

*Kritchevsky, D., et al "Experimental Atherosclerosis in Rabbits fed Cholesterol-Free Diets." Atherosclerosis, 75, 123-7 (1989).

LIE # 27

Animal fat intake leads to atherosclerosis.

FALSE

ANSWER: The International Atherosclerosis Project Report of Autopsy Findings is cited by diet/heart proponents as the most comprehensive and systematic study of post-mortem findings on aorta and coronary atherosclerosis in different populations. The report of autopsies of 31,000 people from 15 countries reported essentially zero correlations between estimated animal fat intake and degree of atherosclerosis or serum cholesterol level.*

*McGill, H.C. Jr. "Introduction to the Geographic Pathology of Atherosclerosis." Lab Invest, 18,465 (1968).

LIE # 28

Vegetarian diets are beneficial for health and vegetarians are said to have significantly lower serum cholesterol levels than non-vegetarians.

FALSE

ANSWER: What is not always reported is that both male and female vegetarians consistently have lower HDL cholesterol levels. Although male vegetarians have lower coronary heart disease than male non-vegetarians, they have equal all-cause mortality. Female vegetarians, on the other hand, have higher coronary heart disease mortality than female non-vegetarians, as well as much higher all-cause mortality. Autopsy studies have indicated that vegetarians have as much atherosclerosis as non-vegetarians even though the vegetarians have lower serum cholesterol levels.*

*Ellis, F.R. et al "Veganism, Clinical Findings and Investigations." American Journal of Clinical Nutrition, 23, 249-255 (1970).

Annual Death Rates for Vegetarians and Non-Vegetarians		
	CHD	All-cause
Male Vegetarians	.22%	.93%
Male Non-vegetarians	.33%	.89%
Female Vegetarians	.14%	.86%
Female Non-vegetarians	.10%	.54%
Data from Burr & Sweetnam, 1982 (Cited in Kato et al).		

LIE # 29

The French diet is higher in total fat and especially in saturated fat and cholesterol than North Americans. French men and women therefore have higher coronary heart disease rates.

FALSE

ANSWER: France is one country that remains an enigma to the proponents of the diet/heart hypothesis. Though the French consume more fat in general and more saturated fat and cholesterol, they have much lower coronary heart disease rates. They have the second lowest rate of the industrialized countries. The French consume more dairy fat. However, they consume much less soybean oil and vegetable shortening. It should be noted that vegetable shortening in the United States are partially hydrogenated and contain substantial amounts of trans-fatty acids. Many of the shortenings in France are not "partially hydrogenated".

The French Diet: What are the differences?		
Source	United States	France
Dairy products **	20.2 lbs.	33.8 lbs.
Vegetable fats & oils	49 lbs.	33 lbs.
Soybean oil	18 lbs.	5 lbs.
Shortening	24 lbs.	4 lbs.
Animal fats (Lard)	2 lbs.	4 lbs.
Total	77.2 lbs.	80.8 lbs.

** Including milk, cheese and butter
* Fat from different sources
* Per person per year, as reported in Hippocrates May/June 1990 (Le Paradoxe Francais Be E. Dolnick) Having been adapted from "The Food Balance Sheet," WHO, 1983, Appropriate calculations added for dairy fats.

LIE # 31

The current standard for a healthy diet is a low-fat, low-cholesterol regimen, which is also known as "The Prudent Diet".

FALSE

ANSWER: These diets promote vegetable oils, high fat crackers, potato chips, peanut butter and margarines. They are advertised as health snacks. The regulatory agencies' acquiescence to these fraudulent health claims are criminal. Their consequences are children who experience growth failure and "Nutritional Dwarfing."*

*Pugliese et al "Parental Health Beliefs as a Cause of Non-organic Failure to Thrive." American Journal of Clinical Nutrition, 43, 622 (1986).

Lifshitz, F. & Moses, N. "Growth Failure: A Complication of Dietary Treatment of Hypercholesteremia."
American Journal Dis Child, 143, 537-42 (1989)

LIE # 32

Cholesterol levels have increased dramatically in the 20th century which caused the epidemic of coronary heart disease.

FALSE

ANSWER: Cholesterol levels have remained the same over the last 100 years.

LIE # 33

Dietary fat consumption since 1900 has increased sharply contributing to the rise in coronary heart disease.

FALSE

ANSWER: The increase in dietary fat over the last 90 years has been trivial. The types of dietary fat have changed. 100 years ago the fats in the diet were more "animal" and more saturated. The major trend since 1915 has been to consume fats with increased polyunsaturation. Since that time our epidemic of coronary heart disease has developed.

LIE # 34

It seems that rule number one to stay in good health is to avoid eating eggs. "Eggs are okay, just don't eat the yolks." The egg white is just as good a source of nutrition as the yolk.

FALSE

ANSWER: Most health professionals are well aware of the high nutrient density of eggs and the broad range of vitamins and minerals eggs contain. What many seem to forget is that the majority of these essential nutrients are concentrated in the yolk. The table below shows that the majority of water soluble vitamins and minerals, all of the fat soluble vitamins, and 45% of the high quality protein are located in that all too often discarded yolk. From a nutritional perspective, this is a prime example of quality nutrition being sacrificed in the name of those dietary demons "fat and cholesterol." So for good nutrition, it is unwise to throw away those yolks because you wouldn't get the full nutritional value an egg has to offer.

Donald J. McNamara Ph.D. Executive Editor Egg Nutrition Center Washington, D.C. "Nutrition Close Up"

PERCENT RDA IN 2 EGGS		
	Whole	White
Protein	21	11
Vitamin K	62	0
Riboflavin	30	17
Vitamin B 12	16	4
Vitamin D	12	0
Vitamin A	12	0
Folate	12	<1
Phosphorus	18	2
Iron	8	1
Zinc	8	<1

LIE # 35

There is a direct association between cholesterol levels and the coronary heart disease death rate.

FALSE

ANSWER: The Framingham Study Experience finds virtually identical death rates for subjects of either sex across a range of cholesterolemia from 205 to 265 mg./dl.

Framingham Data- 30 Year Observation*

Cholesterol mg/dl

Men	205-234	235-265
Deaths per 1000		
Age 35-44	3	6
Age 45-54	11	11
Age 55-64	20	21
Age 65-75	22	23
35-64 Age adjusted	13	14
Women		
Age 35-44	1	1
Age 45-54	4	2
Age 55-64	8	7
Age 65-74	11	13
35-64 Age adjusted	5	4

*Seltzer, C.C. "The Framingham Program Study shows no increases in CHD rates from cholesterol values of 205-265 mg/dl.

G Ital Cardiology, 21, 683 (1991).

LIE # 36

There are many ways to treat high cholesterol levels that are efficacious and safe.

FALSE

ANSWER: There is no treatment of high cholesterol levels known to be both efficacious and safe.*

*Professor James McCormick- "Coronary Heart Disease."

*Thompson, S.G., Pocock, S.J. "The Variability of Serum Cholesterol Measurements: Implications for Screening and Monitoring."

Journal of Clinical Epidemiology, 43, 783-9 (1990)

Mogadam et al "Within Person Fluctuations of Serum Cholesterol and Lipoproteins."

Archive of Internal Medicine, 150, 1645-48 (1990)

LIE # 37

Cholesterol tests can be reproduced and show the same level upon retesting.

FALSE

ANSWER: Cholesterol levels cannot be reproduced. A recent study has demonstrated this truth. Fasting levels of serum cholesterol and Lipoproteins were measured on a weekly basis for four weeks in twenty subjects aged 20-63 years. Variations greater than plus or minus 20% were seen in 75% of the levels of serum cholesterol. On retesting, 40% of the individuals moved from "desirable" to "high risk" category, or vice-versa.*

*Thompson, S.G., Pocock, S.J. "The Variability of Serum Cholesterol Measurements: Implications for Screening and Monitoring."

Journal of Clinical Epidemiology, 43, 783-9 (1990)

*Mogadam et al "Within-Person Fluctuations of Serum Cholesterol and Lipoproteins."

Archive of Internal Medicine, 150, 1645-48 (1990)

LIE # 38

In the early 1900's, people would have had coronaries if they hadn't died of pneumonia or tuberculosis.

FALSE

ANSWER: Today people are dying of heart attacks at ages earlier than most people died of tuberculosis in the early 1900's.

LIE # 39

The epidemic of coronary heart disease was caused by Americans increasing their consumption of animal fats and cholesterol.

FALSE

ANSWER: Animal fat consumption decreased during the so-called epidemic from 1920 through 1989. Animal fat consumption declined from 25 pounds per capita to 10.5 pounds per capita. Vegetable fats increased from 10 pounds per capita to 50.4 pounds per capita, a 500 percent increase.*

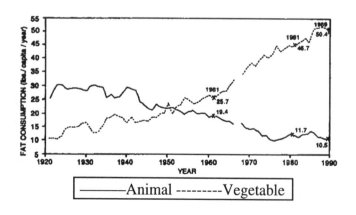

*Kummerow, F.A. Ph.D., "View Point on the Report of the NCEP Expert Panel on Detection, Evaluation and Treatment of High Cholesterol in Adults." Journal of the American College of Nutrition Volume 12, No.1, 2-13 (1993)

LIE # 40

The increase in consumption of vegetable fats is responsible for the decline in heart attack deaths from 1968 through 1988.

FALSE

ANSWER: This is not possible since the same trends have been under way since the beginning of the century, i.e. animal fat consumption has been decreasing and vegetable fat consumption has been increasing.

LIE # 41

The multiple risk factor intervention trial (MRFIT) in 1976 demonstrated a strong relationship between high cholesterol levels and the coronary heart disease death rate. 362,000 men were screened.

FALSE

ANSWER: The coronary heart disease death rate increased from 0.5 to 1.8 per thousand persons per year across the entire range of cholesterol levels. The coronary heart disease death rate increased only (0.13) thirteen one-hundredths of one percent going from the lowest to the highest cholesterol levels. The trivial difference in deaths makes a cholesterol reading meaningless.

LIE # 42

The medical literature presents the picture that there is a strong relationship between cholesterol levels and coronary heart disease death rates.

FALSE

ANSWER: The medical literature is distorted making it impossible to see the true relationship between cholesterol levels and coronary heart disease death rates. Blood Cholesterol does not distinguish between CHD and non CHD for the majority of people. Most people with coronary heart disease have low to moderate levels of cholesterol and most people with high levels of cholesterol do not die of coronary heart disease. These facts are fully acknowledged by prominent members of the research community, the same ones who are responsible for the national cholesterol scare.

LIE # 43

The following statements of fact never made it to the press or other media outlets!

Dr. Scott Grundy, AHA spokesman- "The total number of coronary deaths is greater in the segment of the population with cholesterol levels below 250 mg."

Dr. Mark Hegsted, former director of the USDA nutrition center, "The report of the World Health Organization (WHO) and many others have emphasized that the majority of heart attacks occur in individuals with serum cholesterol levels below 240 mg."

Dr. William Castelli in 1989 reported, "One-half of all heart attacks now occur in people whose serum cholesterol is

225 mg. or less. This means that heart attacks occur equally across all cholesterol levels."

Dr. W.E. Freeman reported "That 66% of male CHD patients had cholesterol levels below 250 mg.."

Dr. Gregory Livshitz pointed out that of the men who died in the MRFIT study, 62% had cholesterol levels less than 240 mg..

LIE # 44

Saturated fat consumption is the real culprit because it increases your cholesterol level which, in turn, causes a heart attack and ultimately, death.

FALSE

ANSWER: This whole cholesterol theory that animal (saturated) fat causes heart disease is fraudulent. The basis of this whole argument by the proponents of the cholesterol myth can be destroyed with the fact that animal fat consumption has decreased since 1900 while the so-called heart attack epidemic was taking place.

LIE # 45

There is a strong association between animal fat consumption and blood cholesterol levels.

FALSE

ANSWER: The International Atherosclerosis Project, published in 1968 stated that while a correlation was found between atherosclerosis and blood cholesterol levels, no association was found between animal fat consumed and blood cholesterol levels. Diets were widely different. Raised arterial lesions were found in virtually all groups by ages 25-34. This study concluded that animal fat was not related to coronary heart disease, a conclusion that is never mentioned by any researchers in their review of this study.

LIE # 46

The American Heart Association and the National Heart, Lung and Blood Institute say you should consume more poultry and fish and less red meat. They say red meats are higher in fat, saturated fat and cholesterol.

FALSE

ANSWER: This statement is absolutely and unequivocally untrue! But the public is brainwashed and poultry is consumed in greater quantities than beef in the American diet. 7.5 ounces of red meat has 145 mg of cholesterol, fish 140 mg. and chicken 186 mg.

LIE # 47

Dietary cholesterol has a profound effect on blood cholesterol levels.

FALSE

ANSWER: This stand is contradicted by the venerable Framingham Heart Study. Only trivial benefits can be obtained by eliminating all cholesterol from one's diet.

LIE # 48

Early studies discovered that vegetable fats, particularly polyunsaturates reduced cholesterol levels. The American Heart Association in 1961 recommended that Americans increase their consumption of polyunsaturates "substantially." This proved to be highly beneficial to humans.

FALSE

ANSWER: Evidence is mounting through the years that polyunsaturated fat is harmful to animals and humans.

LIE # 49

Alcohol consumption increases cholesterol and causes atherosclerosis or clogging of the arteries.

FALSE

ANSWER: It has been known since 1904 that coronary heart disease was less prevalent in the arteries of alcoholics. Two between nations studies showed that the more alcohol consumed by a nation, the lower the coronary heart disease rates, less atherosclerosis and larger diameter arteries were found in drinkers. It takes more than two drinks to raise HDL somewhat and lower LDL somewhat. Total cholesterol remains unchanged. Most reviewers found that some alcohol protects against coronary heart disease. Framingham investigators knew this long ago but withheld publication because of the National Heart, Lung and Blood Institute's long-time stand against alcohol consumption.

LIE # 50

Fish oil supplements lower cholesterol and lead to lower coronary heart disease rates.

FALSE

ANSWER: The increase in America's consumption of fish oil supplements followed a 1972 study of Greenland Eskimos which indicated that large amounts of fatty fish exhibit low rates of coronary heart disease. The fact is that the authors offered no evidence that Eskimos had low coronary heart disease rates. Primitive Eskimos rarely live beyond age 50, long before symptoms appear in the vast majority of people. The study did not indicate the average age of their subjects. This was important. The cholesterol level of the Eskimos was higher than the average American. Studies of other populations in which fish consumption is heavy have found no relationship between fish consumption and either blood cholesterol levels or coronary heart disease rates.

LIE # 51

Cholesterol-lowering trials have proved conclusively that high blood cholesterol levels are directly related to coronary heart disease.

FALSE

ANSWER: There have been more than 30 cholesterol-lowering trials over the last forty years. If the blood-cholesterol relationship is so powerful why should it take so many trials and forty years to confirm it? The truth is that trial after trial failed to confirm it. At least once in every 20 trials by chance alone, some positive findings can occur.

LIE # 52

The lipid research community wholeheartedly believe that high cholesterol levels cause heart attacks.

FALSE

ANSWER: Dr. Robert Levy, National Heart, Lung and Blood Institute Director in 1977, stated before the senate select committee on nutrition, "The problem with all these trials is that none of them have shown a difference in heart attack or death rate in the treated group."

Dr. Basil Rifkind, of the NHLBI, in 1979, said, "To date, no study has actually shown that lowering cholesterol is of benefit in preventing heart attacks."

One NHLBI staff member presented a review of 17 clinical trials at an NHLBI workshop conference and concluded that treatment in these trials did not result in lower overall death rates in any single or combination of trials.

LIE # 53

Lowering cholesterol is beneficial to your health.

FALSE

ANSWER: The overwhelmingly negative findings from 27 clinical trials which used subjects with the highest cholesterol levels indicates that cholesterol-lowering may not have practical benefits for this unique group. There is, in fact, an abundance of proof that lowering cholesterol is harmful to good health.

LIE # 54

Low cholesterol levels can help in preventing not only heart disease but lower the incidence of cancer.

FALSE

ANSWER: On the contrary, 31 studies including Framingham, 7 countries study and the giant multiple risk factor intervention trial (MRFIT) reported higher cancer or total death rates with subject who have lower blood cholesterol levels. Eleven studies found no such relationship. The majority of studies lean toward negative correlations, suggesting that low cholesterol levels may facilitate the growth of cancers or other diseases.*

Rose, G., Blackburn, H., Keys, A. "Colon Cancer and Blood Cholesterol" The Lancet, 1974 1, 523

LIE # 55

Polyunsaturated oils are important because they lower cholesterol levels. In 1961, Americans were advised to replace saturated of animal fats with polyunsaturated or vegetable fats.

FALSE

ANSWER: 1. Diets high in polyunsaturated fats suppress the body's natural immune system. 2. Many researchers have reported evidence linking cancer with a high intake of polyunsaturated fats. 3. Auto-oxidation of polyunsaturated fats contribute to cancer causation. This process involves oxygen and polyunsaturated fatty acids, which result in peroxidation and free-radicals which can cause cells to become cancerous. Japan, Iceland, Norway and Sweden consume the highest intake of polyunsaturated fatty acids from fish and have two to three times the gastric cancer than that of United States males.

Polyunsaturated fats re-saturate when repeatedly heated or exposed to air and become chemical compounds that are similar to varnish, shellac and plastic. One investigator referred to hydrogenated fat as "sheer hard plastic."*

> "Plastic Fat Instead of Butter." Nutrition Health Review Fall 1978, 24.
>
> Encyclopedia notes that polyunsaturated oils become "solid, tenacious films in the presence of air." They are used in the manufacture of paints, varnish and linoleum." Note the similarity of "linoleic" acid and linoleum.*
>
> Gordon, T. "Serum Cholesterol and Heart Disease." Journal of the American Medical Association, 1987, 257, 1600

LIE # 56

The answer to high cholesterol levels is the low-fat, low-cholesterol diet which is currently recommended for all Americans, including children.

FALSE

ANSWER: Cholesterol is vital to the growth of the brain and nerve tissue, and fat is extremely important during the growth process in which high energy is needed. The American Academy of Pediatrics is strongly opposed to the recommendation of low-fat, low-cholesterol diets for children which lead to elevated glucose and insulin levels.

LIE # 57

Fish oil consumption and cholesterol-lowering drugs reduce coronary heart disease mortality.

FALSE

ANSWER: Overwhelming evidence thus far indicates that neither cholesterol-lowering nor consumption of fish oils increases life expectancy or reduces coronary heart disease deaths. The billions of dollars of drugs do more harm than good. "It is like selling the people rope so they can hang themselves."

LIE # 58

Cholesterol-lowering drugs are efficacious although physicians would acknowledge that there are many side effects.

FALSE

ANSWER: In 1987, Dr. Scott Grundy, American Heart Association spokesman stated, "almost all drugs have side effects or the potential for side effects." That is an understatement. The most serious side effect is death. There is evidence that these drugs cause liver changes and cataracts. Recent findings show that they increase LP(A), an unique version of the bad cholesterol. This LDL particle is said to be the true cause of atherosclerosis.

LIE # 59

Alcohol increases coronary heart disease rates.

FALSE

ANSWER: All studies show that alcohol lowers coronary heart disease rates. Most studies 0-3 drinks per day. Some 6-9 drinks per day. The American Heart Association and the National Heart, Lung, and Blood Institute claim more than one drink per day is harmful. A great deal of evidence that 6 shots a day (Linus Pauling) appear beneficial. The warning is that alcoholism leads to cirrhosis of the liver. Dr. Joseph Pursch, The world renowned expert points out that only 11 percent contract cirrhosis.

No one advocates alcoholism, but with the billions spent on research, one physician aptly put it, "Americans should be told that not drinking alcohol is a "cardiac risk factor." Another, "The harmful effects of alcohol occur only at high dose levels."

LIE # 60

Aspirin has significant benefits with coronary heart disease.

FALSE

ANSWER: Nine (9) trials on aspirins were conducted. Seven (7) found no benefits with coronary heart disease or life expectancy. An 8th reported a small reduction. Researchers hailed the last trial as "conclusive." Total all-cause deaths were the same in the aspirin and control groups. There were more strokes. Aspirin is an acid. Regular use can possibly cause bleeding, ulcers, nausea, and vomiting. Adding vitamin C to aspirin can cause stomach damage.

LIE # 61

Cholesterol tests are reliable and reproducible.

FALSE

ANSWER: The accuracy of cholesterol tests are questionable. In 1985, the College of American Pathologists (CAP) sent a blood sample having a known value of 262.6 mg to 5,004 major hospital laboratories (the best in the United States). Values ranged from 101 mg to 524 mg, a 318% difference. The CAP understatement was "between lab reproducibility is not good." 300 million cholesterol tests were performed in 1986 and 1987. A CAP survey in 1988 indicated "about half of the nation's private laboratories regularly return inaccurate cholesterol measurement." Everyone (except the public and the practicing physicians) knows that cholesterol measurement accuracy is exceedingly poor.

LIE # 62

A couple of cholesterol tests should be sufficient to learn the correct level of an individual.

FALSE

ANSWER: Dr. Mark Hegsted called the results of single tests "meaningless." And even a few tests will not be adequate. Dr. Scott Grundy, AHA spokesman agreed that even a series of measurements may not be enough. Dr. Ancel Keys stated, "if you want to be sure within 5%, the test would need to be repeated 5 to 10 times. Millions of tests over the last twenty years have yielded incorrect results. There is no excuse for this senseless activity in the 1990's and beyond.

LIE # 63

The current guideline for high cholesterol is that over 200 mg. is borderline high, over 240 mg. is high. Is this really true? Is the 200 mg. level a proper guideline?

FALSE

ANSWER: In 1984, Dr. Scott Grundy called mild cholesterolemia 225 mg.-275 mg.. Moderate levels were 275 mg.-325 mg.. As late as 1987, the former president of the American Heart Association called more than 260 mg. high cholesterol. The current high level is 85 mg. lower than that defined in 1984. Since the average blood cholesterol is 220 mg., 65 percent of the population will be classified as borderline high or simply high. As the cutoff points have been lowered over the years, so have the revenues of physicians, drug companies, instrument makers, and food producers grown. The National Heart, Lung, and Blood Institute estimated that 40 million people will have high blood cholesterol levels. Cholesterol-lowering drugs will cost up to $3000 per person. The total cost could soar to $10 billion per year by the year 2000. Cholesterol testing and treatment is becoming one of the largest and richest industries in the world.

LIE # 64

The diet/coronary heart disease link is almost universally accepted by physicians and the public at large. Is there truly a relationship between diet and heart disease?

FALSE

ANSWER: Medical literature is alive with evidence which contradicts this concept. Most of the medical scientific community refuses to recognize the flaw in the notion that diet is a major cause of coronary heart disease. The medical establishment has insisted for 62 years of this century that there was a great epidemic caused by an increasing consumption of fats and cholesterol. This hypothesis depends on the assumption that animal fat and cholesterol increased during that period thereby representing the major cause of the epidemic.

All the food consumption trend studies agree that dietary cholesterol did not increase and animal fat consumption steadily decreased during that period. It is well-known by everybody, including the establishment that common sense prevailed and vegetable oils increasingly replaced animal fats throughout this century.

LIE # 65

There is no safe level of cholesterol.

FALSE

ANSWER: The notion that there is no safe level of cholesterol is ludicrous. Cholesterol is an absolutely essential substance in the body. One cannot exist without it. Dr.'s. Raymond Reiser and F.B. Shoreland conclude that "It is unbiological and unreasonable that an essential blood constituent should be toxic at all levels."

LIE # 66

Lowering cholesterol will cause atherosclerosis to regress.

FALSE

ANSWER: It is a fact that vegetarians have coronary heart disease rates equal to non-vegetarians. Since vegetarians already have low cholesterol levels and high CHD rates, it is illogical to believe that atherosclerosis can regress in non-vegetarians by lowering their cholesterol levels either with drugs or by changing their diets.

LIE # 67

The (NCEP) National Cholesterol Education Program recommends the prudent diet for both men and women. Is this necessary for women?

FALSE

ANSWER: The scientific evidence overwhelmingly shows no connection between blood cholesterol and coronary heart disease for women. The two largest studies in the United States and England showed female non-vegetarians had lower coronary heart disease death rates than vegetarians. The most recent statistics suggest no evidence of a coronary heart disease increase for white women during this century. Why are they being told to change their diets and take cholesterol-lowering drugs?

LIE # 68

The American Heart Association and allied entities funded by the National Institutes of Health advocate the Prudent Diet. Is this wise?

FALSE

ANSWER: The Prudent Diet advocated has less than 30% total fat calories and up to 60% of calories from carbohydrates. HDL cholesterol is most important because total cholesterol correlates only weakly with coronary heart disease. Dr. William Castelli recently stated "Cholesterol reading by itself is no clue to a "healthy heart." He maintains that HDL is a more powerful risk factor than LDL...or total cholesterol. The lower the HDL level, the higher the chances of coronary heart disease.

High carbohydrate diets which is what the Prudent Diet really is can "produce some disturbing effects on plasma lipoprotein levels raising VLDL (precursor of LDL) and lowering HDL.*

*Dr. Scott Grundy JAMA 1986, 256, 2823

Thus, the NCEP is advocating a high-carbohydrate regimen that is antagonistic to what is considered to be the "most powerful" protection against CHD. The late Dr. Theodore Cooper, former director of the National Heart, Lung, and Blood Institute, Assistant Secretary of Health, and Chief Executive of the UpJohn Company, (now the Pharmacia and Upjohn Company) stated before Senator McGovern's Select Committee on Nutrition and Human Needs, "But it is true that the consumption of high carbohydrate sources with the induction of obesity constitutes a very serious health problem in the underprivileged and economically disadvantaged." It is precisely this "high carbohydrate diet" that is being promoted with this Prudent Diet. In the 1970's, this "unhealthy" diet was called the "starchy" and is now called "high in complex carbohydrates." But starches and complex carbohydrates are one and the same.

LIE # 69

Cholesterol causes coronary heart disease.

FALSE

ANSWER: The majority of coronary heart disease patients have low to moderate levels of cholesterol and most people with high cholesterol levels do not die of CHD. Thus, some factor other than cholesterol must be responsible for CHD development. Until such factors are discovered, it is best to attribute coronary heart disease (CHD) to genetic predisposition.

LIE # 70

An American Heart Association study showed that diet was responsible for coronary heart disease.

FALSE

ANSWER: In the 1950's, the American Heart Association contracted with a group of researchers to review all diet-coronary heart disease data. The group included Dr.'s. Irvine Page, Frederick Stare, H.C. Corcoran, Herbert Pollack, and Charles Wilkinson.

In 1957, they published a very thorough and objective report. They suggested that an epidemic of coronary heart disease may not have occurred during this century. They noted that the American diet had not changed during this century in ways that the idea that dietary cholesterol or fats could be responsible for the so-called epidemic.

The American Heart Association buried the report for four years, and in 1961, a "revised" and "updated" report was published. The AHA statement omitted the most important findings presented in the 1957 report, the two conclusions in the preceding paragraph. Three of the first report's authors were replaced. Two of the replacement authors (Ancel Keys and Jeremiah Stamler) were fully committed to the belief that a coronary heart disease epidemic had taken place and that it was due to changes in the American diet. Not only was the 1961 statement an improper derivation of the 1957 report, it was slightly more than two pages, and had 23 references. How could it be "updated" or "revised" when the original version was twelve and one-half pages and had 87 references?

LIE # 71

Animal fat derived from red meat is the culprit in heart disease. A diet which is low in fat and cholesterol can prevent coronary heart disease.

FALSE

ANSWER: Dietary cholesterol remained constant throughout this century (Randall and Slattery 1988) and Call and Hansen stated "Few Americans seem to be aware of the fact that they have derived a higher proportion of their fat from plant sources and less from animal sources since the turn of the century."

During the period in which the reported coronary heart disease mortality rate increased the most (1950-1962), egg

consumption in the United States decreased 18 percent
(Medical World News 11/13/89).

LIE # 72

Cholesterol clogs coronary arteries.

FALSE

ANSWER: After 30 years of examining coronary heart
disease patients and thousands of bypass procedures, world-
famous surgeon Michael DeBakey reported no association
between cholesterol levels and artery occlusion.

LIE # 73

High density lipoprotein (HDL) cholesterol, the so-called
"good" cholesterol is more important in preventing coronary
heart disease than total cholesterol levels.

FALSE

ANSWER: Not only is the relationship between the HDL
level and coronary heart disease equally as weak as that
between total cholesterol and CHD, HDL is difficult to raise
and it is almost impossible to measure accurately in most
laboratories across the country. In fact, in 1988 Dr. Bernadine
Healy (American Heart Association president) warned
physicians not to emphasize HDL cholesterol because it is
difficult to increase in the bloodstream. Dr. James Cleeman
said "If low HDL is the problem, we don't know what to do
about it." The National Heart, Lung, and Blood Institute said
there is no "sure method of raising HDL levels."

LIE # 74

Risk factors for heart disease are smoking, high blood pressure, and high cholesterol levels. There are many others such as sex, obesity, and lack of exercise. Most Americans believe that high cholesterol levels lead to coronary heart disease.

FALSE

ANSWER: All risk factors have no predictive value. The research community does not publish data that only 28 percent of the population dies of coronary heart disease. (We can therefore guess correctly 28 percent of the time). This fact is further evidence that blood cholesterol level alone has a very weak predictive value.

LIE # 75

Most Americans who are over 50 years of age must monitor their cholesterol level and keep it under 200 mg./dl with diet, exercise, and if necessary, cholesterol-lowering drugs.

FALSE

ANSWER: In 1977, the famous Framingham Heart Study reported in the Journal of the American Medical Association (JAMA) that there was no significant correlation between cholesterol and coronary heart disease for persons over 50 years of age. While this is widely known in the medical literature, it is doubtful that it is known to physicians and the lay public.

LIE # 76

Total cholesterol levels are not as important as HDL (high density lipoprotein) levels in the development of coronary heart disease.

FALSE

ANSWER: Not only is the relationship between the HDL level and coronary heart disease equally as weak as that between total cholesterol and coronary heart disease, HDL is difficult to raise and it is almost impossible to measure accurately in most laboratories across the country. In fact, in 1988, Dr. Bernadine Healy, (then president of the American Heart Association) warned physicians not to emphasize HDL cholesterol because it is difficult to increase in the bloodstream. Dr. James Cleeman said, "If low HDL is the problem, we don't know what to do about it." The National Heart, Lung, and Blood Institute's Dr. Basil Rifkind said "There is no sure method of raising HDL levels."

LIE # 77

Risk factors such as high cholesterol levels, high blood pressure, and smoking have a strong predictive value for coronary heart disease.

FALSE

ANSWER: A condition, substance, or behavior that has been associated with coronary heart disease but has not been proven to cause the disease is known as a "risk factor." Smoking, Blood pressure, and cholesterol are risk factors for coronary heart disease. 200 risk factors have been proposed by researchers. The American Heart Association and the National Heart, Lung, and Blood Institute recognizes 11 risk factors including age, obesity, sex, and lack of exercise. However, all of the risk factors have almost no predictive value. The researchers do not publish data that 28% of the population dies of coronary heart disease. In other words, we can guess correctly 28% of the time. This fact is further evidence that blood cholesterol level alone has a very weak relationship with coronary heart disease.

To better focus on how meaningless risk factors are, Dr. Herbert Naito states that "Among individuals undergoing bypass surgery at the Cleveland Clinic Foundation, about 35% demonstrate none of the known risk factors except a hereditary predisposition to the disease. For most persons with CHD, however, we observe at least one of the major risk factors predominating. 35% show no major risk factor, 65% show at least one.

LIE # 78

In the years 1912-1960, when food technologists learned how to transform perishable vegetable oils into solid, storable margarines, the politically powerful dairy industry suppressed margarine marketing by bringing about restrictive regulations and taxation. Then, in 1961, with the release of the American Heart Association "Dietary Recommendations", the tables were turned. Partially hydrogenated vegetable fats were touted as protectors and animal fats such as butter and lard were put down as causing coronary heart disease. Is the AHA recommendation valid?

FALSE

ANSWER: Vast fortunes were made in the vegetable oil industry. The John Hopkins Medical School has an

Anderson-Clayton research building sponsored by the Anderson part of Anderson-Clayton, a major vegetable oil company. But when polyunsaturated oils are hydrogenated, a new kind of fatty acid is produced. These "trans-fatty acids cause quick and dramatic increases in cholesterol levels when fed to human subjects.* One of the widely promoted hydrogenated spreads which claims "heart protection" is Fleischmann's margarine. It contains 24% trans-fatty acids. Why do the FDA and FTC allow this travesty to continue?

*Mensink, R.P., Katan, M.J. "Effect of Dietary Trans-Fatty Acids on High Density and Low Density Lipoprotein Cholesterol Levels in Healthy Subjects."
New England Journal of Medicine, 323, 439 (1990)

LIE # 79

Americans are bombarded with health claims in food advertising and packaging. Foods are touted as cholesterol-free and therefore "heart savers." Can the public be confident that these claims are true?

FALSE

ANSWER: Ancel Keys, who is a pioneer in the evolution of the diet-heart-cholesterol hypothesis, wrote in the New England Journal of Medicine in 1991, "Dietary cholesterol has an important effect on the cholesterol level in the blood of chickens and rabbits, but many controlled experiments have shown that dietary cholesterol has a limited effect in humans."*

For 36 years, we have been witness to a distortion of science. Keys had become unimpressed with the results of his own seven countries study and other investigations. Why else would he express a statement so profoundly opposite to his position for the last 36 years.

*Keys, A., Letter "Normal Plasma Cholesterol in a Man Who Eats 25 Eggs a Day." New England Journal of Medicine, 325, 584 (1991)

New York Times-July 14, 1987 Boffey, P.M. "Cholesterol Debate Flares Over Wisdom in Widespread Reductions."

LIE # 80

The clinical trials sponsored by the National Institutes of Health have yielded conclusive proof that dietary cholesterol leads to high blood cholesterol levels and subsequently to atherosclerosis, heart attack, and death.

FALSE

ANSWER: There have been 33 trials of the diet-heart hypothesis in the last 30 years. The evidence consistently says, "No-this is not a sound hypothesis." These trials have failed to prove the theory they were unfortunately undertaken to prove. The dilemma we now face is a consequence of human frailties. We hold on to the disproven hypothesis because of "pride, profit, and prejudice." How can those little people admit they have made such a dreadful error? How can the American Heart Association admit its error? Its fund-raising program would self-destruct. There's no turning back for those in power. How can the bureaucrats go before a congressional committee and admit they wasted billions of taxpayer dollars for research? These people are entangled in a web of deception that has worked toward the detriment of the American public.

LIE # 81

The buildup of cholesterol on the arterial wall of man is the only logical cause of atherosclerosis with the inevitable result of coronary heart disease.

FALSE

ANSWER: The pathology of atherosclerosis in man and the experimental production of the disease from the initial intimal proliferation in stock-fed herbivorous animals merely by altering the blood flow support the concept that atherosclerosis is a hemodynamic disease and that the disease develops irrespective of the blood cholesterol level. Variation in severity within the species depends on genetically determined and individualistic biochemistry, vascular topography, cardiovascular physiology including blood pressure and individual variability in response to physical and emotional stress. Obviously culture, race, stature, nutritional status, and coexistent disease may contribute indirectly to the variation in severity from person to person, but it would be wrong to place equal or greater emphasis on such secondary factors and thus detract from the important role of hemodynamic stress. Exception may be taken to such a mechanical concept of the etiology and pathology of atherosclerosis, but vibrational stress with fatigue failure provides a logical explanation for the origin of the disease, which cannot be accounted for by the lipid hypothesis.

Finally, it must be concluded that hemodynamic stress not only localizes but can cause initial intimal proliferation and the progression to overt atherosclerosis and its complications without the presence of hypercholesteremia.*

Stehbens, W.E. M.D., *Stehbens, W.E. Experimental

Induction of Atherosclerosis Associated with Arterio-venous Fistulae in Rabbits on a Cholesterol-Free Diet 1991. Submitted for Publication.

LIE # 82

The Center for Science in the Public Interest (CSPI) vigorously promotes the dogma of the American Heart Association and the National Heart, Lung, and Blood Institute. In late 1986, tropical oils were targeted as a "cardiovascular time bomb". The result was a campaign by the soybean industry to replace tropical oils (which are saturated) with soybean oil. This was a wise decision which was definitely beneficial for the heart health of the public.

FALSE

ANSWER: Before their removal from food, tropical oils represented 4% of the fat in a typical American diet. This amount is trivial. The change amounted to 1 milligram of cholesterol. What is more, the fats used to replace the tropical oils are hydrogenated vegetable oils adding trans-fatty acids to the American diet. While tropical oils were a minor contribution of saturated fats to the American diet, the trans-fatty acids are much more harmful and cause free-radicals that lead to coronary heart disease.

LIE # 83

The average person in America is convinced that cholesterol is the "universal demon" and is to be avoided at all costs. Low-fat low-cholesterol diets are the order of the day, and eggs are a no-no because they are high in cholesterol. This regimen is the right way to go.

FALSE

ANSWER: The major clinical trials were conducted in the United States, Britain, Scotland, and Mainland Europe. The American and British trials were well designed and conducted and almost all of their findings were negative. One reviewer put is this way: "No amount of squirming on the hook alters the fact that no effects of treatment were found."

The overwhelming failure of the trials to provide evidence supporting the presumed benefits of lowering blood cholesterol was compounded by the fact that they were maximally designed to generate such evidence. Males were used in all the trials, while females were used in only 8. This biased results toward greater coronary heart disease incidence. Of the 23 trials, the average initial blood cholesterol levels were 265-266 mg.. These levels were higher than their respective populations. Therefore, if lowering cholesterol is beneficial, it should have been most demonstrable in these subjects.

LIE # 84

Saturated fat increases your cholesterol level and causes heart disease.

FALSE

ANSWER: After reviewing the dietary factors observed in Israel, McMichael*1 concluded that "polyunsaturated fat does not prevent coronary heart disease, and might even be suspected of contributing to its development."

Blondheim*2 reported that experience in Israel cast doubt on the assumption that "eating a low-fat diet with a high ratio of polyunsaturated to saturated fatty acids protects against coronary heart disease." The Israeli experience showed that as immigrants increased their intake of vegetable oil their serum lipids were increased and coronary heart disease increased as well. The Bedouins in Israel, who had been eating animal fat in the desert began eating vegetable fat as they moved into the towns, and then their problems with coronary heart disease began.

*1 McMichael, J. "Fats and Atheroma: An Inquest" British Medical Journal, 1, 173-175, 1975

*2 Blondheim, S.H. "Polyunsaturation of the Diet and the Development of Ischemic Heart Disease."
Talk given at the MacDonald College of McGill University, 5 October, 1983

LIE # 85

Exercisers believe that vigorous and even punishing exercise leads to better health and longer life. They feel that cardiovascular health is promoted by exercise and protects against heart attacks, the leading cause of death.

FALSE

ANSWER: The medical profession has played a major role in the exercise revolution, providing a legitimacy where there otherwise would be none. But not every physician who recommends exercise does it solely for profit. Doctors themselves participate in vigorous workouts. They are consumers like everyone else and subject to the same ballyhoo and hype as the rest of the population.

This amazing exercise phenomenon, fueled by the profit

motive and supported by a population worried about its health, has a terrible momentum. The sober truth may not stop it, but it should be stated. You may enjoy exercise, it may help you socially, you may look and feel better, but all the rest is myth. "Exercise will not make you healthy. It will not make you live longer. Fitness and health are not the same thing."

Fitness is measured physiologically by oxygen consumption. This doesn't mean a thing to your heart. Running conditions the muscles, but does nothing for the lungs. If cardiovascular health was a product of physical training, then fit people wouldn't die of heart disease. The fact is that exercisers suffer the same ills that plague us all. The leading cause of exercise-related deaths in well-trained people is coronary heart disease. You can be fit and healthy. You can also be physically fit and ill with coronary heart disease. Finally, you can be unfit and unhealthy as well.

> Henry A. Solomon M.D. "The Exercise Myth". 1984
> From a review in "The Best of Health" 1990, Sheldon Zerden

LIE # 86

A press release for the LRC-CPPT trial (Coronary Primary Prevention Trial) stated that "in summary the LRC-CPPT is the first study to demonstrate conclusively that the risk of coronary heart disease can be avoided by lowering blood cholesterol."

FALSE

ANSWER: The fact is that coronary heart disease deaths over 7.4 years were as follows: There were 38 deaths in the control group and 30 deaths in the drug group. The CPPT results were withheld from the public. However, in statements to the medical community, the National Heart, Lung, and Blood Institute's Dr.'s. Claude Lenfant and Basil Rifkind stated, "It has to be recognized that evidence linking diet to coronary heart disease, however compelling, will always fall short of certainty."

Lawrence Friedman, Chief of Clinical Trials Branch of the NHLBI recently observed that, "There is no such thing as a definitive clinical trial. The results of a clinical trial alone are not necessarily persuasive, nor should they be." These statements are light years apart from the LRC-CPPT authors' press release.

Some investigators emphasized that the LRC study offered no proof that modifying diet will lead to a reduced risk of coronary heart disease. Many expressed concern over the increase of genitourinary cancers and other diseases in the drug treated group.

Another writer summarized the results as follows: "Despite a determined effort on the part of the LRC-CPPT to convince the public that at long last we now had the answer to the cholesterol problem, the results were disappointingly unconvincing."

It is probable that the authors' preconceived opinions and the expenditure of $150 million of public funds were too great for the LRC investigators to conclude that anything less than outstanding success was achieved.

LIE # 87

Authors of the Helsinki trial concluded that it provided "additional and conclusive evidence" that lowering blood cholesterol prevents coronary heart disease. Dr. Basil Rifkind made the same pronouncement, "The outcome of the Helsinki Heart Study is conclusive."

FALSE

ANSWER: Such lavish praise was not warranted for another trial which failed to demonstrate a difference in total deaths between groups. In fact, the treatment group suffered a slightly higher overall death rate.

The drug used in the study, Gemfibrozil, is similar to Clofibrate, which was found to be ineffective in three previous clinical trials. Finally, it should be reemphasized that the Helsinki trial was entirely funded by Warner Lambert, maker of the drug Gemfibrozil. The trial represented a "significant" part of the $177 million invested in Gemfibrozil. Obviously Warner Lambert would not be pleased if the authors reported negative findings with such a large investment.

LIE # 88

The sharp decline in the cardiovascular death rate which started in 1964 was "attributed to the improvements in nutrition and serum cholesterol as well as other risk factors."[1] "In part, to the decrease in cholesterol concentration of the general population."[2]

FALSE

ANSWER: Food trends were the same as they were before coronary heart disease rates declined, and most studies indicate that blood cholesterol levels have not changed much if at all during the last 40 years. For example, Dr. Ancel Keys obtained an average value of 219 mg. for 541 men in 1949. Dr. William Kannel reported an average of 220 mg. for his Framingham men in 1971. The largest distribution of cholesterol ever obtained, the Multiple Risk Factor

Intervention Trial (MRFIT) showed an average cholesterol of 215 to 220 mg. in 1973-1975. And in 1988, Dr. Herbert Naito reported the average value to be 220 mg..

*1 Kannel, W.B. "Twelve Questions Frequently asked by Physicians" Consultant 1988, 28, 25

*2 Naito, H.R. "New Cholesterol Consciousness Outlook for Aggressive Management" Physician's Marketplace, 1987

LIE # 89

Your cholesterol level can never be too low. The lower the better.

FALSE

ANSWER: There is a danger in reducing blood cholesterol. Population studies reported the relationship between blood cholesterol and cancer. 32 studies have shown higher cancer rates at lower cholesterol levels. The 1989 analysis of the MRFIT data showed a sharp upturn in mortality at low cholesterol levels.

It has been known for decades that cholesterol protects cells from toxic substances. It is not surprising that low levels of blood cholesterol may promote such disease as cancer. When asked by New York Times reporter Gina Kolata about the relationship between low cholesterol levels and cancer, Dr. Salim Yusuf replied, "I can't fully explain it and it worries the hell out of me!"

Dr. William Kannel neglected to tell his readers that he had previously reported (1983) that lung and colon cancer rates were higher in men with cholesterol levels under 190 mg. than with levels greater than 190 mg.. He also reported that breast cancer rates were higher among women with lower cholesterol levels.

LIE # 90

Treating high blood pressure with drugs leads to lower coronary heart disease death rates.
FALSE

ANSWER: There have been controlled studies which showed that subjects treated for high blood pressure with drugs exhibited higher coronary heart disease death rates than those not treated. Dr. Kannel's 30 year Framingham data revealed that heart attacks were on the increase during that period for both people with normal blood pressure and those who were being treated for high blood pressure. Dr. Kannel said that these findings "suggest that the previously reported adverse effect of diuretic (drug) therapy was not a factor." But rather than emphasize that the drug caused no harm, Dr. Kannel should have emphasized the more important information, namely, that the lowering of high blood pressure by drugs had no health benefits.

LIE # 91

The advice of all experts is to reduce consumption of dietary cholesterol from 600 mg. to 300 mg. a day.

FALSE

ANSWER: "I disagree with the well-meaning advice of prestigious organizations that recommend a reduction of dietary cholesterol consumption from 600 mg. to 300 mg. a day. I disagree because such a reduction would result in a less nutritious diet for most people; it would not prevent human atherosclerosis. The calories supplied by eggs, meat, and milk would probably be replaced by low-protein, high-fat food items with the possibility that more rather than less calories would be consumed. Sufficient high-protein vegetable food items at less cost and the equivalent value to eggs, meat, and milk are not available. The low-calorie foods which are recommended as a replacement for animal protein foods are expensive and not as "satisfying" as high-calorie foods such as soft drinks, potato chips, french fries, and candy bars. The result may well be a diet higher in fat and more deficient in protein, vitamins, and minerals, thus facilitating more rather than less atherosclerosis."*

Kummerow, F.A. "Nutrition Imbalance and Angiotoxins as Dietary Risk Factors in Coronary Heart Disease" The American Journal of Clinical Nutrition, January 1979

LIE # 92

The total serum cholesterol among Chinese varies between 150-160 mg./dl. This would help prevent coronary heart disease.

FALSE

ANSWER: The leading cause of death in Beijing is Cerebral Vascular Disease (also due to atherosclerosis) followed by cancer and coronary heart disease. The Chinese who consume more whole grains and vegetables and less milk, meat, and eggs have a life expectancy 10 years less than Americans or Europeans.

"Has China Failed?" New York Review 1979, 26, 33

LIE # 93

If you watch your diet, avoid cholesterol and saturated fat, give up smoking, and keep your blood pressure under control, the chances are good that you can extend your life for many years.

FALSE

ANSWER: In a review of data obtained from a number of epidemiological studies (Taylor et al 1987) constructed a model to provide quantitative data for an increase in life expectancy if one adhered to a lifelong "prudent" diet. Be their calculation, a non-smoking, normotensive, 40 year old male with an average cholesterol level would increase his life expectancy by 10 days.

LIE # 94

Most dietary clinical trials show reduction in heart disease and total mortality in those people who were on a low-fat, low-cholesterol regimen.

FALSE

ANSWER: The public is unaware that in most tests which showed a reduction in death rates from coronary heart disease, the total mortality was not decreased. Most people are also not aware that in a number of studies total mortality actually increased in the group who were on a low-cholesterol, low-saturated fat diets compared to those persons on high-cholesterol, high-saturated fat diets.*

*Chris Mudd "Cholesterol & Your Health-The Great American Rip-off" P.18

LIE # 95

The largest government sponsored dietary trial conclusively proved that changes in your eating habits would lower your blood cholesterol and thereby prevent coronary heart disease.

FALSE

ANSWER: The Multiple Risk Factor Intervention Trial or MRFIT was one of the most demanding medical experiments ever performed on human beings. It took ten years, involved 28 medical centers across the nation, employed 250 researchers, and cost $115 million dollars.

361,662 men aged 35 to 57 years of age were screened to get 12,866 men who were at high risk from multiple factors. Two-thirds smoked cigarettes, two-thirds had high blood pressure. Their typical diet contained twice the recommended amount of cholesterol. The candidates were divided into two groups. One was given the "usual" care by their doctors. The other "special" intervention group underwent a campaign to change their living habits. The subjects made extensive changes in their eating habits, reducing dietary cholesterol, saturated fats, and overall calories. The changes had little effect in the level of their blood (serum) cholesterol. Blood cholesterol dropped only 5 percent by one measurement and 6.7 percent by another. The study had a modest goal of 10 percent.

The researchers expected to reduce the coronary heart disease deaths by 25 percent. On February 28, 1982, more than 9 years after the experiment started, they tallied the results. The trial was a complete failure. There was no significant difference in the overall number of deaths between the two groups. In fact, slightly more deaths occurred in the special intervention group. The major surprise was a 40 percent lower number of deaths from coronary heart disease in the usual care group.

LIE # 96

At about the same time as MRFIT was underway, a new trial called the CPPT or (Coronary Primary Prevention Trial) was launched. A drug called Cholestyramine (Questran) was used to interfere with normal digestion. The researchers expected to reduce cholesterol 50 percent in the treatment group.

FALSE

ANSWER: The liver produces bile acid which circulates through the intestine, where it breaks down fats into a more usable form. Investigators believed that Cholestyramine attacked the LDL (or bad cholesterol) and they expected the drug to reduce the total cholesterol by 25 percent and the LDL even more.

Half the subjects received the drug, and half a placebo. It was therefore a double blind study. Diet was also part of the study (which was expected to achieve a 3 to 4 percent cholesterol reduction). After 7 years, coronary heart disease would have been reduced by 50 percent in the treatment group. 480,000 middle-aged men were screened. 3,810 subjects were found in 3 years. The subjects had extremely high levels of cholesterol, higher than 95 percent of the population. Men 35 to 59 years of age were used because they had a greater risk of heart attack. This unusual group which was especially vulnerable, increased the odds of success in an expensive and demanding experiment. Both the placebo and the drug caused severe side effects and there were fears that because 68 percent of the subjects reported side effects of gas, heartburn, and bloating, that many of them would drop out.

The results after 7 years were disappointing. The cholesterol levels in the treatment group were only 6.7 percent lower than those in the control group. This was 25 percent of the expected drop. So—this lengthy, expensive, $142 million dollar trial was a failure. It could not decisively prove the hypothesis. The study did prove one thing..that the body has an effective mechanism for maintaining blood cholesterol levels.

LIE # 97

The World Health Organization (W.H.O.) Set out to prove that the drug Clofibrate could lower blood cholesterol and achieve a 30 percent reduction in coronary heart disease.

FALSE

ANSWER: After five years, the study in three European countries made it obvious that blood cholesterol could only be lowered by 9 percent. The group taking Clofibrate had 162 deaths compared to the control group's 127 deaths with the same cholesterol levels.

Clofibrate caused gallstones, cancer, and affected the liver and the digestive system. In sum, the cholesterol-lowering drug seems to have killed more people than it saved. Instead of accepting this failure, heart institute researchers continued their quest for a test that would confirm their predetermined result. This is completely unscientific.

LIE # 98

Salt intake should be lowered to prevent high blood pressure.

FALSE

ANSWER: A major international research project in 32 nations showed that while the incidence of Hypertension varied widely, salt intake had little to do with it. The human body has a powerful mechanism to maintain a specific level of dissolved salt in the bloodstream and quickly eliminate any surplus. Therefore normal adult consumption of salt can vary over an extremely wide range without altering the internal balance.

LIE # 99

Dr. Jeremiah Stamler maintained that "The International Atherosclerosis Project in its final report includes a valuable chapter on the relationship of nutrition to the disease. A highly significant correlation was found between the intake of fat and atherosclerosis at autopsy."

FALSE

ANSWER: In fact, no correlation between animal fat (saturated) intake and either degree of atherosclerosis or blood cholesterol level and concluded that the type of fat was not related to coronary heart disease.*

Yet Dr. Stamler maintained that the project provided evidence that "A cause and effect relationship has been demonstrated between dietary lipids (specifically saturated fat and cholesterol) and widespread premature coronary heart disease." He neglected to say that the project didn't report any association between coronary heart disease of blood cholesterol and animal fat, by far the major source of saturated fat and a significant source of cholesterol.

*Scrimshaw, N.S. & Guzman, M.A. "Diet and Atherosclerosis" Laboratory Investigation 1968, 18, 623

LIE # 100

Northern Indians eat a high-cholesterol, high-saturated fat diet. Southern Indians eat 44 percent polyunsaturated fats. The Northern Indians have a higher incidence of heart disease.

FALSE

ANSWER: The fact is that the Northern Indians, who eat lots of animal fats, butterfat, and milk do not have more heart disease. The Southern Indians who have a low-cholesterol diet have 15 times more heart disease than the Northern Indians with the high-cholesterol diet. Better nutrition explains the difference. These results have not been widely publicized.

LIE # 101

The majority of people with serum cholesterol of 222 mg. or higher develop coronary heart disease.

FALSE

ANSWER: The truth is that only 20 percent of heart disease patients have serum cholesterol levels above 222 mg. Dr.

Michael DeBakey quoted in the Washington Star, June 15, 1972 said, "Much to the chagrin of my colleagues who believe in this polyunsaturated oil and cholesterol business, we have put our patients on no anti-cholesterol medications. About 80 percent of my 1,700 patients with severe atherosclerosis requiring surgery have cholesterols of normal people." Dr. DeBakey is perhaps the most well-known heart surgeon in the world.

LIE # 102

A diet of saturated fat, dairy products, and eggs will lead to a higher incidence of heart disease.

FALSE

ANSWER: In Japan, there was a 14 percent decrease in heart disease since 1955 while their diet has increased in dairy products, eggs, and saturated fats.*

"Supernutrition" Richard Passwater Page 74

LIE # 103

People with high cholesterol levels usually have atherosclerosis (clogged arteries).

FALSE

ANSWER: Many people with high cholesterol levels have no signs of atherosclerosis.

LIE # 104

Genetics is the primary cause of coronary heart disease.

FALSE

ANSWER: If that is true, why was there such an increase in deaths from coronary heart disease between the mid 1920's and 1968? Did our genes change in a matter of a few decades?

Chris Mudd-Introduction of "Cholesterol and Your Health"

LIE # 105

If you correct risk factors, you can prevent, retard, or reverse coronary arteriosclerosis.

FALSE

ANSWER: A principal architect of the Framingham Heart Study, which established coronary risk factors, has declared *1 "There are few prophylactic measures of proved efficacy in coronary heart disease. This applies to primary and secondary prevention. Neither hygienic, pharmacological, nor surgical measures have been shown to delay acute episodes or prolong life."

"So far, despite all the effort and money that have been spent, the evidence that elimination of risk factors will eliminate heart disease adds up to a little more than zero in terms of preventing heart disease on a public health scale."*2

*1 Kannel, W.B. "Prevention of Coronary Heart Disease by Control of Risk Factors" Questions and Answers
Journal of the American Medical Association 227:338, 1974

*2 "Can I Avoid a Heart Attack? Lancet 1:605, 1974

LIE # 106

Cholesterol-lowering drugs are beneficial in lowering the incidence of coronary heart disease.

FALSE

ANSWER: The Food and Drug Administration has demanded that advertisements for certain lipid-producing drugs carry this qualifying codicil: "Important Note: It has not been established whether drug-induced lowering of serum cholesterol and other lipid levels has a detrimental, a beneficial, or no effect on morbidity or mortality due to atherosclerosis or coronary heart disease."

LIE # 107

Vigorous exercise can reverse arteriosclerotic lesions and decrease the danger of death from coronary heart disease.

FALSE

ANSWER: The National Heart, Lung Institute stated in 1971, "The idea that regular physical exercise decreases the danger of death or disability from coronary atherosclerotic disease is based on a number of assumptions, some proven and some of questionable validity. But, there is no convincing data to indicate that exercise will, in fact, decrease either the rate of development of atherosclerosis, or prevent its complication."*

*National Heart and Lung Institute task force on arteriosclerosis: "Arteriosclerosis: A Report by the

National Heart and Lung Institute Task Force on Arteriosclerosis-National Institutes of Health, Vol 11-Washington D.C. U.S. Gov't Printing Office-June 1971

LIE # 108

Cholesterol is the major risk factor for coronary heart disease.

FALSE

ANSWER: Dr. Lars Werko, a World Health Organization scientist, in observing the Framingham statistics remarked, "It seems, therefore, rather remarkable when looking at the results regarding deaths...that there is not any straight line relation between the level of serum cholesterol and the incidence of these deaths."*1

Dr. Werko further stated, "Nevertheless, the most active epidemiologists working in this field emphasize the importance of serum cholesterol___or high blood lipids__ as the risk factor. Many want, therefore, to recommend far-reaching dietary measures in order to control the blood lipids in the population as the most important preventive measure against coronary heart disease.

It is, then, rather surprising to find the following statement from the Framingham Group: "In the balance, blood pressure appears to be the strongest of the factors considered for coronary heart disease and atherothrombotic brain infarction. For either clinical event there appears to be little difference in the strength of this factor from one age group to another."*2

*1 American Heart Journal January, 1976, Vol.91, No. 1 pp.87-98

*2 CIBA Symposium 12: Atherogenesis: Initiating Factors, New York, 1973 Elsevier

LIE # 109

Polyunsaturates lower cholesterol and prevent heart disease.

FALSE

ANSWER: The fact is that there is more evidence to show that polyunsaturates cause disease rather than prevent it. Recent studies have linked an intake of more than 10% polyunsaturates to vitamin deficiencies, premature aging, liver damage, nutritional muscular dystrophy, severe blood diseases in infants, and cancer.

A 1975 study in American Laboratory by C.E. West and T.G. Redgrave reports that a group of infants fed a formula with a high content of polyunsaturates developed skin lesions and blood changes associated with vitamin E deficiencies. Vitamin E supplements caused these conditions to disappear.

In a Mayo Clinic study, it was shown that patients who had breast cancer also had an increased amounts of polyunsaturates in their breast tissue and their blood plasma. In an 8 year study on two groups of men at the Veteran's Hospital in West Los Angeles, one group was given four times as much polyunsaturated fatty acid as the other group. It was found that those on the increased polyunsaturates diet had 60% more cancers than those on a regular balanced diet. The study was publicized in 1971.

A polyunsaturated fatty acid is more unstable than an unsaturated fatty acid because it has an even greater number of reactive atoms in its molecule. It is the oxidation of polyunsaturates due to their instability, that produces the harmful effects in the body. When polyunsaturated fats oxidize, they produce extremely toxic lipid peroxides. The heating of polyunsaturates further increases toxicity by causing them to form polymers__the chemical compounds that produce plastics, varnish, and shellac__and the longer a polyunsaturated oil is heated, the more dangerous it becomes. (Think of this when you order French Fries that have been fried in stale restaurant grease that has been heated for hours on end)

"The Cholesterol Controversy" authors Dr. Ed Pinckney and Cathey Pinckney report: "That polyunsaturates form varnish in the body was demonstrated when animals that were fed such heated fats were found the next morning stuck to their cage floors by their varnish feces. Some of the animals suffered total intestinal obstruction from the polymerized polyunsaturates. When animals were fed heated polyunsaturates and heated butter to note the effect on their health... all of the animals given heated corn oil developed tumors, and only one of the original 96 survived the 40-month experimental period. In contrast, none of the animals fed heated butter developed tumors and all survived."

All of the facts concerning polyunsaturated oils should be a warning to the Americans who are eating them at a rate 500% higher than in 1920* see table 1. The consumption of animal fats has dropped sharply over the last 70 years, and all this was happening while the so-called heart disease epidemic was sweeping the country.

LIE # 110

The AMA Council on Foods and Nutrition has recommended that "Members of the media and publishers as well as authors of books and articles advising the public on diet and nutrition have a unique responsibility to ensure that such information and advice are based on scientific facts established by responsible research." Physicians share a similar responsibility. The American Heart Association has been careful to exercise scientific due diligence in its advice to the public.

FALSE

ANSWER: With this awesome responsibility in mind, let us examine the recommendations and publications of the American Heart Association and the Inter-society Commission for Heart Disease Resources. Knowing full well that there is no scientifically established proof that lowering serum cholesterol by either diet or drugs will prevent atherosclerosis, the Inter-society Commission, composed of "outstanding leaders in the field of cardiovascular disease and representatives of national professional organizations capable of making a significant contribution" has cleverly circumvented this debatable point. In addition to other advice of questionable value as to dietary changes, they recommended a reduction of egg yolk consumption, not because it has been proven harmful, but because it "will seriously hamper dietary programs aimed at reducing cholesterol." Consequently, the public should be encouraged to avoid egg yolk consumption, and the food industry should be persuaded to minimize egg yolk content of commercially prepared foods."*

Unfortunately, this advice by the commission and other groups antedating the commission has succeeded in reducing American egg consumption; because the housewife does not differentiate between egg yolk and whole eggs. She hears the message that eggs are not good for you, therefore she buys no more eggs for her family. Despite the drastic reduction of egg consumption (30-35%) and a similar decrease in whole milk intake, the epidemic of heart attacks has continued and expanded.

*Stamler, J. et al: "Primary Prevention of the

Atherosclerotic Diseases." In report of the Inter-society Commission for Heart Disease Resources Ed. By Wright, I.S. and Frederickson, D.T. Circulation 42: 1970 Revised April 1972.

LIE # 111

The consumption of animal fats (saturated) increases cholesterol and is responsible for the atherosclerotic lesions which lead to a heart attack.

FALSE

ANSWER: The International Atherosclerosis Project* found that "available data regarding dietary consumption were not sufficiently precise to determine whether type of fat and amount of cholesterol in the diet are important in relation to atherosclerosis. The estimated percentage of total dietary fat consisting of animal fat does not appear to be associated with severity of atherosclerosis."

*McGill, Fr. H.C. Editor: The Geographic Pathology of Atherosclerosis. Williams & Wilkins Baltimore, 1968

LIE # 112

Polyunsaturated fats lower cholesterol and prevent atherosclerosis.

FALSE

ANSWER: "The ignorance inherent in the recommendation to avoid dietary cholesterol is paralleled by the ignorance in the recommendation to add unsaturated fatty acids to the diet in order to reduce serum cholesterol. No scientific evidence exists to support the contention that eating increased amounts of polyunsaturated fats prevents atherosclerosis, but there is definite scientific evidence from animal experiments that a glut of polyunsaturated acids causes or accelerates potential cancer due to possible formation of benzopyrenes and peroxides. This has never been shown for saturated fats. Populations on fat-poor diets, such as the Japanese, have a high incidence of stomach cancer, a fact omitted from the reports emanating from the American Health Foundation."*

*Oster, Dr. Kurt A. "The Decline of Common Sense and the Ascent of Computerized Nonsense in Medicine. Journal of Applied Nutrition - 1975.

LIE # 113

Coronary heart disease death rates declined 27% in the United States from 1968 to 1977. Surgeon General Julius Richmond reported that per-capita consumption of milk, cream, eggs, and butter had fallen significantly since 1965. Milk and cream declined 21%, eggs 10%, and butter 28%. It would then follow that the lower rate of saturated fat consumption influenced coronary mortality.

FALSE

ANSWER: Whether diet is a major factor in the coronary heart disease death rate decline is debatable. Switzerland has experienced a major, long-term decline in deaths from all types of heart disease despite a concurrent rise of 20% in animal-fat consumption. In Japan, the already-low coronary death rate continues to fall, although intake of saturated fats has soared 200 percent.*

*Consumers Union Report May 1981

LIE # 114

The National Cholesterol Education Program (NCEP) guidelines for cholesterol control states that under 200 mg. is desirable, 200-239 mg. Is borderline high, and over 240 mg. Is high. Does this guide to what is considered a good cholesterol level take an individual's age into consideration?

NO!

FALSE

ANSWER: Anyone versed in the biology of aging knows that serum cholesterol increases with age. The older you get the higher your cholesterol level. The Inter-society Commission is mainly a creation of the American Heart Association. Science recognizes no manifestos; it aspires to the truth. The commission's report frightened the American people. It frightened them with the data on the death rate of atherosclerotic disease "which was propaganda, and a reservoir of half-truth." Dr. Kurt A. Oster stated, "I have examined some of the statistics expounded by the Inter-society Commission and found them to be false, distorted, and not even corresponding to the original source material."*1

Knowing full well that there is no scientifically established proof that lowering cholesterol will prevent atherosclerosis "Outstanding leaders in the field of cardiovascular disease and representatives of national professional organizations capable of making a significant contribution" failed in their scientific duty. In addition to other advice of questionable value as to dietary changes, they recommended a reduction of egg yolk consumption, not because it has been proven harmful, but because it "will seriously hamper dietary programs aimed at reducing cholesterol."

Let us heed the message contained in the first annual report of the National Heart and Lung Advisory Council in 1974.* "We do not know how to prevent atherosclerosis or how to diagnose and treat it early and we tend to obscure our ignorance by making it seem that a program has been solved." We must face up to our ignorance in many matters and recognize that an entirely different type of knowledge than we now have will be necessary to fully solve these problems.

It is interesting to see the age-related cholesterol guide issued by the National Heart and Lung Institute in 1974.*2

Table of concentrations of cholesterol which if exceeded clearly indicates Hyperlipidemia *3

Age	Mg. Per 100 ml.
1-19	230
20-29	240
30-39	270
40-49	310
50-	330

*1 Oster, K.A. "Prevention of Atherosclerosis-Fact or Fiction? Medical Counterpoint 4:No. 4 1972

*2 First Annual Report of National Heart and Lung Advisory Council July 29, 1974 U.S. Gov't Printing Office, DHEW Pub. No. (NIH) 74-508

*3 The Dietary Management of Hyperproteinemia National Heart and Lung Institute DHEW Pub. No. (NIH) 75-110 Reprinted 1974

LIE # 115

It is no secret that eggs contain a great deal of cholesterol, and many doctors recommend that their patients eat only the white of the egg. The reason is obvious. Eggs increase your cholesterol and could be a factor in causing heart attacks and strokes.

FALSE

ANSWER: Dr.'s. Cuyler Hammond and Lawrence Garfinkel of the American Cancer Society conducted a study on the dietary habits of 804,409 persons who had no previous history of heart disease or stroke. After a six-year period, 14,819 of these had died of heart disease and 4, 099 had died of stroke. These subjects were divided into two groups at the inception of the study. The first group consisted of those who ate whole eggs five or more times a week in addition to the eggs consumed in the preparation of other foods. The second group ate fewer than four eggs per week or no eggs at all. (The American Heart Association now recommends no more than four whole eggs a week). Those in the second group who ate practically no eggs had more deaths from heart attacks and strokes than those who ate all the eggs they wanted.*

*Passwater, Richard Ph.D. "Supernutrition" The Dial Press-1975 Page 68

LIE # 116

A low-cholesterol diet is effective in preventing heart disease.

FALSE

ANSWER: One of the many studies which disprove the myth of a relationship between dietary cholesterol and coronary heart disease is a study at the University of Minnesota. A low-cholesterol diet was fed to thousands of persons for four and one-half years. It showed that the low-cholesterol diet was of no significant help in preventing heart disease. Dr. Ivan D.

Frantz of the university stated, "I still believe in the theory but it's awfully hard to demonstrate. It may be that over a lifetime a low-cholesterol diet would be of some benefit."

The survey was reported at the 48th scientific sessions of the American Heart Association, involving 17,000 patients of state hospitals in Minnesota. This "captive" group was chosen so the their diet could be strictly controlled. "In the entire population, including men and women of all ages over 21, despite a satisfactory decrease in blood cholesterol, there was not the slightest hint of benefit," Dr. Frantz reported.

Autopsies of the patients who died during the study showed no difference in the amount of atherosclerosis (clogged arteries), no matter which diet was eaten.

"State Study Casts Doubt on Links Between Heart Attack, Cholesterol." Minneapolis Tribune Tuesday November 18, 1975 AP

LIE # 117

The level of cholesterol in the blood of children is directly related to the cholesterol in their diet.

FALSE

ANSWER: Dr. William Wiedman reported in Anaheim, California to a scientific session of the American Heart Association. He found that fatty food may not be the culprit in high blood cholesterol levels. In a 3-year Mayo Clinic study of more than 2,500 school children, Dr. Wiedman showed that high blood cholesterol levels may not be linked to diet.

"Our study in children reveals no significant importance between levels of cholesterol in their blood and what they eat." A team of five Mayo Clinic investigators conducted the project which was financed by a $2.1 million dollar National

Institutes of Health grant.

"There was no correlation between the level of cholesterol in the blood and the amount of cholesterol in the food they ate," Wiedman said. Some who ate less cholesterol had higher levels of cholesterol in their blood than those who ate foods high in cholesterol. Wiedman said the next logical step would be a more comprehensive investigation "from birth to about age 21."

"Study Finds No Fat Link to Children's Cholesterol"
The Minneapolis Star Wednesday, November 19, 1975

LIE # 118

Cholesterol and Triglyceride levels are dependent on the consumption of fat, sugar, starch, and alcohol.

FALSE

ANSWER: Serum cholesterol and triglyceride levels among Americans are much more dependent on the degree of adiposity (obesity) in each person than on his or her consumption of fat, sugar, starch, or alcohol. Therefore weight reduction should be the first step in Hyperlipidemia.

This finding is based on a prospective dietary survey of 4, 057 adults in Tecumseh, Michigan, done by Dr. Allen B. Nichols and Associates of the University of Michigan. The frequency of consumption of 110 different foods was determined for each participant, and the average weekly consumption rates of foods high in fat, sugar, starch, and alcohol were compared with serum cholesterol and triglyceride levels in each person. Lipid levels were also compared with individual adiposity indexes, which included measurements of skin fold thickness.

Serum cholesterol and triglyceride values were not correlated with the frequency of consumption of dietary constituents. However, serum cholesterol and Triglyceride concentrations were positively and significantly correlated with the adiposity index in both men and women.*

*Nichols, Allen B. M.D. Ravenscroft, Catherine MNS, Lamphiear, MA, and Ostrander, Leon D. Jr. M.D. University of Michigan, Ann Arbor "Independence of Serum Lipid Levels and Dietary Habits" Journal of the American Medical Association:236: 1948-53, 1976. Modern Medicine February 1, 1977

LIE # 119

The hysteria surrounding cholesterol and eggs has resulted in a frenzy to develop an egg substitute which retains the nutritional value of the original. Egg Beaters ® provide high quality protein and is cholesterol-free. They are nutritious and meet the growth requirements of the cholesterolphobic public.

FALSE

ANSWER: Egg Beaters ® contain the following according to the label: "Egg white, corn oil, nonfat dry milk, emulsifiers (vegetable lecithin, mono and diglycerides and propylene glycol monstearate), cellulose and xanthan gums, trisodium and triethylcitrate, artificial flavor, aluminum sulfate, iron phosphate, artificial color, thiamin, riboflavin and vitamin D." A comparison of the nutrients in 100 GM. of Egg Beaters ® with the nutrients in 100 GM. of "Farm Fresh Eggs" (Table 1) indicates a list of nutrients which should be able to meet the growth requirements of weanling rats.

Table 1

Comparison of nutrients in Egg Beaters® or shell eggs with the nutrient requirements of growing rats.

Nutrients	100 GM. Egg Beater®	100 gm. of egg	Req. of growing rat
Protein	11	12.8 GM.	13.3 GM.
Fat	12.5	11.4 GM.	5.5 GM.
Calories	166.66	160	G/E day 76 per rat (444 K Cal/100 GM.)
Ca (Mg)	81.6	54	560 mg.
P (Mg)	71	204 mg.	440 mg.
Na (Mg)	181	122 mg.	60 mg.
K (Mg)	213	128 mg.	200 mg.
Iron (Mg)	1.8	2.2 mg.	38.9 mg.
Cholesterol (Mg)	<1.6	550 mg.	--
Vitamin A (Unit)	1.350	1.180	.67 mg. (Retinol/Kg)
Vitamin D (Unit)	43	50	111.1 (I.U/Kg)
Thiamine (Mg)	.13	.1 mg.	.14 mg.
Riboflavin (Mg)	43	.3	.28 mg.
Choline Chloride	*	382 mg.	83.3 Mg/100 GM.
Ca Pantothenate	*	2.7 mg.	.89 Mg/100 GM.
Vitamin B 6	*	.3 mg.	.78 Mg/100 GM.
Vitamin B 12	*	.001 mg.	.00056 Mg/100 GM.
Biotin	*	.04 mg.	.1 Mg/100 GM.

*Not listed

A test was conducted to determine the nutritional value of Egg Beaters® as compared to shell eggs. One group of weanling rats were fed Egg Beaters® and the other was fed fresh whole eggs. 100 shell eggs at a time were cracked into a Hobart Mixer and 125 GM. Of calcium acetate was added and blended for two minutes and stored at minus 20 degrees centigrade until ready to thaw and feed. Six cartons of Egg Beaters® were thawed, 25 GM. Of calcium acetate was added and blended for two minutes in a Hobart Mixer. Both mixtures were stored in a refrigerator, poured into 4 ounce glass jars and fed daily. The calcium acetate was added to meet the recommended nutritional requirement for calcium. Both the mothers and the pups fed Egg Beaters® developed diarrhea within one week; those fed whole eggs did not develop diarrhea. The pups fed the two egg mixtures were weaned at 5 weeks of age. All of those fed Egg Beaters ® died within 3 to 4 weeks after weaning. The general appearance of the rats fed Egg Beaters ® indicated a gross deficiency in one or more nutritional factors. (Figure 1).#1

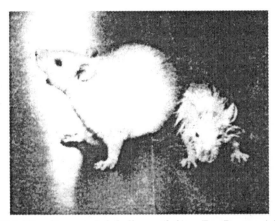

FIG 1. Weanling rats fed shell eggs (left) or Egg Beaters (right).

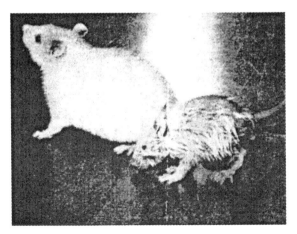

FIG 2. Weanling rats fed shell eggs (left) or Egg Beaters (right). (Both animals were washed with mild detergent, rinsed and dried with paper towels before picture was taken.)

Neither Egg Beaters ® or shell eggs serve as a single food source in the human diet. Furthermore, both Egg Beaters ® and shell eggs were fed in the raw state to see whether Egg Beaters ® has the "nutrition of Farm Fresh Eggs." It is evident that shell eggs which contain the Lipotropic-laden egg yolk, furnish one or more nutritional factors which are absent in Egg Beaters ®. These nutritional factors are no doubt present in the common food items which comprise the diet of human adults and could probably be added to the Egg Beaters' ® formulation.

Following the publication of this study, the Fleischmann Laboratories, Standard Brands, Incorporated changed the formula of the original Egg Beaters ®.*2

*1 Kummerow, Fred, A. Ph.D. & Avidi, Meena Kasmii, M.S. The Burnsides Research Laboratory, University of Illinois Urbana, Illinois 61801 Pediatrics Vol, 53 No. 4 April 1974

*2 Personal Communication from Fred A. Kummerow Ph.D. to Sheldon Zerden

LIE # 120

The National Cholesterol Education Program (NCEP) recommends eating a pat of margarine seven times a day. Ostensibly the panel still believes that the vegetable oils in margarine protect the public from the scourge of coronary heart disease.

FALSE

ANSWER: The truth is that partially hydrogenated vegetable oils in margarine is the primary source of trans-fatty acids that are so detrimental to the integrity of the arteries. Dozens of studies have implicated that substance in the development of coronary heart disease.

The most well-known of those studies, The Harvard Nurses Study of 85,000 people found that people who eat margarine have a 66 percent greater chance of heart disease than those who don't eat food that containing partially hydrogenated vegetable oils.

LIE # 121

Network television advertising commercials and four-color print advertising in the country's largest circulation publications recommend a high-fiber diet to remove cholesterol and its by-products from the body and prevent heart disease.

FALSE

ANSWER: A team of researchers at the University of Oregon Health Sciences Center in Portland, Oregon respond with a resounding "No Way!" In a recent study, the team found that adding crude fiber to high-or low-cholesterol diets had no effect whatever on plasma cholesterol concentrations of the eaters. And though the fiber cut the intestinal transit time, confirming previous work, it did not change cholesterol absorption by the body.

Dr. Thomas L. Raymond, Research Fellow at Oregon concluded that, "Our message is that fiber will not protect a person against coronary heart disease, those who claim that a high-fiber diet protects primitive peoples from cardiovascular disorders often fail to point out that this diet is also low in fat, low in cholesterol, low in meat, low in refined carbohydrates, and low in caloric density. A diet may indeed help prevent heart disease but not by the action of fiber alone."*

*Medical World News February 21, 1977

LIE # 122

Lowering cholesterol by any means will extend your life.

FALSE

ANSWER: The use of cholesterol-lowering drugs in one of the largest and most significant studies showed that more people who were treated died sooner than those who weren't treated. The results from the Helsinki Study (Journal of the American Association, 1991; 286: 1225-1229) After following the study group for 15 years, showed that the death rate from heart disease among the people who were given drugs exceeded the death rate among the drugless group by 242 percent.

LIE # 123

Cholesterol intake correlates directly with the incidence of coronary disease in men aged 55-59 years.

FALSE

ANSWER: Connor and Connor (Preventive Medicine 1: 49, 1972) presented data tending to correlate cholesterol intake with coronary disease. The United States showed the highest cholesterol intake and the highest death rate. Finland had the second highest death rate with a cholesterol intake half of ours. France had a cholesterol intake slightly higher than Finland's but a death rate that was 79% lower.*

*Letter from David Kritchevsky, Ph.D., Associate Director of the Wistar Institute, Philadelphia, PA. To Senator George McGovern's Senate Select Committee on Nutrition and Human Needs. May 24, 1977

LIE # 124

Millions of Americans are now convinced that by avoiding meat, eggs, and dairy products and consuming polyunsaturated fats, they will reduce their chances of becoming victims in the heart disease epidemic that strikes one million Americans annually.

FALSE

ANSWER: The cause of atherogenesis (hardening of the arteries) and heart attacks is still not known. There is no direct scientific proof in humans that eating high cholesterol foods raises serum (blood) cholesterol and no direct scientific proof that high cholesterol leads to heart disease or that lowering the cholesterol reduces the risk of heart disease. Consuming large quantities of polyunsaturates to lower cholesterol may be dangerous.

Perhaps as doctors watch in dismay as their patients on strict low-cholesterol diets suffer heart attacks, it will be concluded that our cholesterol obsession has sidetracked us from pursuing a scientifically broad and objective approach to research into heart disease.*

*Town & Country Article by Nancy Lyon January 1977

LIE # 125

It is a well-known fact that dietary fiber in the form of bran lowers blood cholesterol.

FALSE

ANSWER: The use of bran as a cholesterol-lowering agent was widely recommended in the professional and lay press.

In 1975, it might have seemed that bran should be added to all diets by FIAT. The results of ten publications on the effects of bran on serum lipids in man were collated by Truswell and Kay (Lancet 1: 367, 1976). In a rare show of unanimity nine out of the ten studies found no effect on serum cholesterol levels. The tenth detected a modest (7%) reduction.*

*Letter from David Kritchevsky, Ph.D., Associate Director of the Wistar Institute, Philadelphia, PA. To Senator George M. McGovern's Senate Select Committee on Nutrition and Human Needs May 24, 1977.

LIE # 126

The plaque in human arteries is loaded with cholesterol.

FALSE

ANSWER: An editorial in the Lancet in the October 14, 1978 issue, the subject was "Virus Infections in Atherosclerosis." In this editorial, it was stated that much human atheroma contains little or no cholesterol. It also ended with "The overwhelming emphasis placed on cholesterol in atherogenesis has diverted effort away from other lines of research for nearly two decades."

A world-wide study by Strong et al[1] showed the same degree of atheroma in all parts of the world.

At the University of Washington Earl Benditt used an electron microscope to examine the atheroma of normal patients. He found that it is made up of collagen fibers and of smooth muscle cells that have proliferated out of the media and into the intima of the artery. He calls this "Monoclonal Proliferation.[2]

[1] Strong et al "Laboratory Investigation, Vol. 18, No. 5. May 1968 P. 527

*2 Benditt, Earl P. Ph.D., "The Origin of Atherosclerosis." Scientific American, Feb. 1977, pp. 74-80

The Cholesterol Paradigm

The public has swallowed the orthodox line that cholesterol clogs your arteries and ultimately leads to a heart attack. There is no controversy. It is a fact. Just ask your physician. If your cholesterol level is high, you are cautioned to eat a low-fat, low cholesterol diet. This means you must avoid eggs, bacon, beef, whole milk, butter, ice cream, and hard cheeses.

The diet of our forefathers was a healthy, wholesome, and nutritious regimen that was never known to cause heart disease. In the period since World War I there has been an enormous increase in smoking, sugar consumption, and food processing. This wholesale change in our diet over the last 75 years is responsible for the degenerative disease epidemic which we have today.

The fear of cholesterol has never been more a part of America than it is today in 1997. The orthodoxy has done its job well. The cholesterol paradigm or belief system is so imbedded in the psyche of the public that it is tantamount to a religion. There is no way that you can change the current mind set of individuals who have been bombarded with misleading advertising day in and day out. Why is it necessary to claim that a dry breakfast cereal has "no cholesterol." It is obvious that the buzzword means that it is good or healthy if it contains no cholesterol and bad if it has cholesterol.

Most doctors suggest that cholesterol and fats should be reduced in the diet. They are following the popular, modern, mindless, rush toward nutritional Armageddon. It makes no nutritional sense to exclude from our diet those foods which contain the most wholesome, healthy, and nutritious foods. Millions of people have fanatically avoided foods containing cholesterol at the insistence of their physicians. The tragic irony is that their nutrition-free regimen is actually causing the heart disease it was designed to prevent.

There are societies which eat low-fat diets and still have heart disease, and others that eat high-cholesterol diets and are free of heart disease. The American diet has changed radically from that of our forefathers. They ate bacon, eggs, gravy, whole grains, fresh whole milk, and fresh vegetables. They did not have any heart disease. Cynics have claimed that the reason for the non-existence of heart attacks in the early years of the 20th century was that people were dying of tuberculosis and other contagious diseases at a young age. The truth is that hundreds of thousands of our young men are dying of heart attacks at an earlier age than their counterparts in the early 1900's were dying of contagious disease. What's more, people did live to advanced ages as far back as the late 1800's and didn't suffer heart attacks.

The Cholesterol Myth

The cholesterol myth represents the greatest swindle in the history of nutrition. If you read the paper or watch television, you probably believe the following:

1. Cholesterol is some kind of fat.
2. You get all the cholesterol from the food you eat.
3. Cholesterol causes heart attacks.
4. A healthy diet contains no cholesterol.

The truth is that:

1. Cholesterol is not a fat. It is a solid alcohol.
2. Each day you manufacture 3 times as much cholesterol as you can possibly consume in your diet.
3. About 80 percent of patients with heart attacks have normal cholesterol levels.
4. Cholesterol is an essential part of human metabolism. If you don't include it in your diet, your body will manufacture it for you.

Margarine is the big money-maker promoted by the food industry to replace butter and avoid consumption of cholesterol. It is a 10 billion dollar business. What the "Food Engineers" don't tell you is that margarine does not lower your cholesterol levels and that you are not getting the polyunsaturated oil that is promised in their ads. In order to turn this "pure liquid polyunsaturated oil" into a solid bar of margarine, hydrogen is bubbled through a tank of oil. This hydrogenation hardens the oil into saturated fat. This means you are paying for polyunsaturated fat and getting something like lard. "You might as well cut the fat off your steak and spread it on your toast in the morning!"

The High-Cholesterol Diet

It has never been proven that an elevated level of blood (serum) cholesterol is the cause of a heart attack. Billions of research dollars and decades of studies later, Americans are still dying of coronary heart disease at an alarming rate.

The major organizations which control the research and disseminate their results have bought in to the theory (and it's still just a theory) that dietary cholesterol and saturated fats raise the blood cholesterol, which results in coronary heart disease, and ultimately death. That scenario sounds plausible. It is also very logical. The only trouble is that it doesn't work!

The diet which our forefathers ate at the turn of the 20th century was a highly nutritious, whole food, unprocessed, high-cholesterol diet. There was no epidemic of heart disease then, and most premature deaths were the result of infectious diseases. The study of nutrition was in its infancy and it was not through the application of good nutritional principles that the population avoided heart disease on a grand scale. It was because of a highly nutritious diet. The very foods which our doctors tell us to avoid today...eggs, beef, milk, butter, bacon, cheese etc. were the mainstays of the healthy diet in the early 1900's.

It wasn't until 1913 that Casimir Funk coined the term vitamine. It was the beginning of the science of nutrition. About that time, steel roller mills were invented. They stripped the germ and the bran out of the wheat to produce a pure, refined white flour. While this process prolonged the shelf-life of all products made with the flour, it effectively removed all of the nutritional value of the wheat. The Vitamin E in the germ and fiber in the bran are vital for a highly nutritious diet. Furthermore, it has been said that a fly would not waste its time eating a roll or a piece of white bread. Obviously, the common house fly is smarter than we humans.

America's low-fat, low-cholesterol diet has been

promoted and approved overwhelmingly by most established health organizations, led by the powerful and influential American Heart Association. The National Heart, Lung, and Blood Institute which targets cholesterol as the culprit in coronary heart disease, and diet as the reason for high blood (serum) cholesterol levels endorses the diet, and so does the American Medical Association and most of its members.

So there is no fear that cholesterol levels will increase, and the epidemic of coronary heart disease will continue. Right? Wrong! After a decade or two of decreases in the incidence of heart attack deaths, there is a strong resurgence in the rate of CHD fatalities. This is true despite the fact that there has been no trend of increased cholesterol levels in the population. Therefore, the increased death rate can hardly be blamed on cholesterol.

The consumption of eggs, beef, milk, butter, cheese, and other nutritious, cholesterol-bearing foods have been eliminated from the average American's diet. It has not decreased cholesterol levels, and it certainly has had no effect on the death rate from coronary heart disease, stroke, cancer, diabetes, and other degenerative diseases. It seems that the warning of Dr. Carl Pfeiffer has been ignored, and nutritional Armageddon awaits over the horizon.

Cholesterol Facts

1. Diet does not increase your blood (serum) cholesterol.
2. Saturated fat does not increase your blood (serum) cholesterol.
3. Cholesterol does not cause heart attacks.
4. 80% of people who get heart attacks have a normal cholesterol level. Only 20% of heart disease patients have serum cholesterol levels above 222 mg% (JAMA 1964).
5. Reducing cholesterol intake or reducing blood (serum) cholesterol levels does not reduce the incidence of heart disease.
6. Eggs do not increase your cholesterol level.
7. Controlling heart disease risk factors does not reduce the incidence of heart disease.
8. There is no direct evidence that dietary cholesterol causes heart disease.
9. Low cholesterol diets do not prevent coronary heart disease.
10. High cholesterol diets do not cause coronary heart disease.
11. Low cholesterol diets can increase the incidence of coronary heart disease.
12. Low cholesterol diets can possibly increase the incidence of cancer.
13. The generations that ate gravies, fatback, whole grains, and fresh vegetables did not experience coronary thrombosis.
14. Milk and eggs are two of our best and most nutritious foods.
15. If margarine prevented heart attacks, our heart attack rate would only be one-third its present level since two-thirds of all families regularly use margarine.

16. The American diet has increased its polyunsaturated oil content, and heart disease has paralleled it. In 1989, per capita consumption of vegetable fats was 50.4 pounds per year and animal fats was 10.5 pounds per year. In 1920, animal fats per capita was 26 and vegetable fats was about 11.

17. When a person reaches 50 years of age, cholesterol begins to decline as a risk factor. It continues until at age 65 or 70, it is no longer a risk factor at all.

18. In those instances where diet or drugs lower cholesterol levels, the mortality rate is identical with those who do not diet or take drugs.

19. Low cholesterol readings below 180 have shown an increase in the incidence of cancer.

20. A high blood (serum) cholesterol is a risk factor for heart disease. It is not a causal factor.

21. High blood pressure, obesity, genetics, smoking, stress, and a sedentary way of life are the main risk factors that result in a heart attack.

22. Linus Pauling states that 3 to 4 grams of cholesterol are produced in the body every day.

23. The 20th Century increase in heart disease mortality rates was not caused by cholesterol.

24. Margarine does not lower your cholesterol level.

25. If you lower your cholesterol level you will not increase your longevity.

26. 33 diet-heart trails failed to prove that a high cholesterol diet causes coronary heart disease.

27. Cholesterol levels have remained the same in the United States for the United States for the last 100 years.

28. The consumption of vegetable fats has jumped more than 500 percent since 1920.

29. Americans eat about 3 pounds of sugar and other caloric sweeteners a week. If you add refined flour

and starches the amount increases to 4 pounds a week.

30. Poultry has more cholesterol than beef. 7.5 ounces of red meat has 145 mg., chicken has 186 mg., and fish has 140 mg.

31. 31 studies have shown that low cholesterol levels cause cancer.

32. Dr. William C. Taylor et al, in a government funded survey, found that a 40 year old male with an average cholesterol, who adheres to a lifelong "prudent" diet, doesn't smoke, has normal blood pressure, would increase his life expectancy by 10 days.

33. 40 years of study at Framingham showed "no increased overall mortality with either high or low cholesterol levels among men after age 47." The same is true of women after age 47 or under age 40. "Cholesterol and Total Mortality."

34. From the end of World War II until 1963 mortality from coronary heart disease rose sharply and steadily. Then it declined steeply through the 1970s and 1980s. One factor can be ruled out — cholesterol.

35. Drugs lower your blood cholesterol. While they might have reduced the incidence of heart attachks, they have not improved life expectancy at all.

36. If cardiovascular health was a product of physical traiing, then fit people would not die of heart disease.

37. The cholesterol levels of Chinese is between 150-160 mg./dl. The leading cause of death in Beijing is cerebral vascular disease (due to atherosclerosis) followed by cancer and heart disease.

38. Northern Indians eat lost of animal fats. Southern Indians eat a low-fat, low-cholesterol diet. The Southern Indians have 15 times more heart disease.

39. Polyunsaturated oils (partially hydrogenated fats) accelerate potential cancer due to possible formation of benzopyrenes and peroxides.

40. Across the entire range of cholesterol levels (150 mg. to 350 mg.) the coronary heart disease death rate increased only (0.13%) or thirteen one-hundredths of one percent. This trivial difference in deaths makes a cholesterol reading meaningless.*

*The multiple risk factor intervention trial (MRFIT).

The Food Engineers

We are on the whole a nation of nutritional illiterates. Without assessing blame for our condition, it is obvious that we are committing nutritional suicide. Mountains of potato chips and oceans of cola drinks are only a small example of our cavalier disregard for proper nutrition. The food industry is content to offer those products which the public loves without regard to their nutritional value. Sugar and salt and cholesterol-containing fats and oils abound in every type of processed food artifact whether it is canned or frozen. Processors are more concerned with shelf-life than nutrient content. It starts and ends with money. The public doesn't care. Nutrition doesn't sell. We are well on our way to a nutritional Armageddon.

Our educational system is sorely lacking in many things, but none are more important than the management of our diet. Not only is nutrition not part of the curriculum in the public schools, but it is not even a mandatory subject for medical students. If doctors are going to dispense information to their patients, it is vitally important for them to learn all they can about the biochemistry of man.

Good health is not a gift bestowed upon everyone who is born into this world. It is a goal toward which we all must strive, and a thorough knowledge of the science of nutrition is a great asset. Don't look to your physician for guidance in proper nutrition. You will be told to eat a balanced diet and get enough exercise, and you'll be all right. How many people eat a balanced diet? What is a balanced diet? Are vitamin and mineral supplements necessary? What is the right amount of vitamin C and vitamin E?

When Louis Pasteur convinced the medical world that bacteria caused the infectious diseases of his day, the seeds of orthodoxy were sown. The medical system of today is overwhelmingly drug-oriented, and concentrates on curing illness rather than the prevention of disease. Heroic medical care will always be with us, but no amount of drugs will cure the underlying problem for which they are prescribed. It will be the task of the individual who sincerely cares for his own well being to educate himself in the field of nutrition. In recent years, it has become fashionable for the aware individual to supplement his diet with those vitamins and minerals that are essential to good health. If only a small percentage of the money that is spent on drug research was invested in the search for the nutrients that energize our immune system, that fortify our cardiovascular health, and create the environment that will enhance our skeletal and nervous systems, health care costs can be reduced to an insignificant amount. It is estimated that in the year 2000, the cost for health care will be in excess of one trillion dollars.

The number one killer in America is heart disease. It is variously estimated that about 1,000,000 deaths are caused by heart attacks and strokes every year. Heart attacks are the result of an occlusion or blockage of the coronary arteries which supply the heart with the blood and oxygen to support its function. Strokes are caused by an interruption of the blood flow into the brain. The epidemic of heart disease is a very recent phenomenon. In fact, Dr. White, who was President Dwight D. Eisenhower's physician, could not even study cardiology when he was in medical school. There was no cardiology department in his school. The obvious reason was that heart disease was not a factor in the mortality statistics at turn of the century. It is logical to conclude that the diet of Americans of that era was not causing the scourge which faces us today. The degenerative disease epidemic of cancer, heart disease, diabetes, etc., is a plague of our own design. In the early 1900's, people in The United States had not even heard of the word "cholesterol" and it is safe to assume that they were eating bacon, ham, beef, butter, eggs, whole milk, and many other foods that contain a great deal of cholesterol. Did physician's warn their patients to avoid these high-cholesterol foods? Certainly not. The reason simply is that those foods which contain cholesterol are the most nutritious foods you can eat. Not only are they necessary for good health, but depriving yourself of their beneficial nutrients can render you nutritionally deficient and lead to all sorts of debilitating physical and mental conditions. The irony of today's consensus of using a low-fat, low-cholesterol diet to prevent coronary heart disease is that you may actually be causing the condition that you are trying to prevent!

How do we as intelligent human beings approach the problem of diet, nutrition, and longevity?

1. We must agree that health is our #1 problem and responsibility.
2. Assume that good nutrition prevents disease.
3. Learn all we can about the science of nutrition.
4. Pledge to ourselves not to eat anything that is known to contribute to the deterioration of our health.
5. Diligently maintain the proper attitude toward good health and nutrition.
6. Realize that our commitment to good health must last a lifetime.

Nutrition Nightmare

America is a nutritional nightmare. It is a bomb waiting to explode! Dr. Carl Pfeiffer, the late head of the Brain Biocenter in Princeton, New Jersey stated in his book, "Mental and Elemental Nutrients," "We are headed for nutritional Armageddon!"

It has been estimated that 50 million Americans are obese. It cannot be argued that all this overweight can be caused by genetics. It is more likely to be an omnivorous national binge that disregards the most elementary rules of good nutrition.

The soft drink industry is now a $64 billion dollar industry. Ice cream is at least a $10 billion dollar business, and the cookie business is about an $8 billion dollar business. In total, the food service industry is now a $600 billion dollar business, and it is growing larger every year.

At the root of this march to disaster is the total lack of any nutritional knowledge by the public. This tragedy has evolved because our educational system fails to teach the fundamentals of healthy eating. To add to the problem, our medical schools rarely have any mandatory courses in nutrition. How can our doctors hope to give us dietary advice without a trace of biochemical experience.

It is understandable that our medical practitioners do not care to learn about nutrition that would prevent disease. Their business is almost exclusively prescription medicine. They treat the symptoms of disease and not the cause. This unfortunately results in continuous treatment with drugs which have side effects and do not cure the underlying problem.

The answer to America's nutritional disaster is education. Doctors and individuals must educate themselves on the subject of nutrition. The information is out there. If we ignore the rules, we are subject to the inevitable penalty...poor health, sickness, and premature death.

Cholesterolphobia

Cholesterolphobia is epidemic in America. It has taken three decades for the fear to sink deeply into the subconscious of the masses. The initial suspicion that high blood cholesterol was a leading factor in the development of atherosclerosis (artery disease) was reported in the early 1950's. The "Lipid Hypothesis" was unproven in the accepted scientific approach to disease but the temptation was too great to resist. The medical profession, the food industry, the pharmaceutical industry and the government agencies which are charged with the responsibility of finding the answer to our health problems embraced the theory as though it were fact.

Throughout the decades following World War II, the incidence of heart attack death rose in a straight line until it became the number one killer in the nation. The public wanted answers and it was convenient for the medical community to lay the blame on cholesterol. Doctors told their patients to stop eating eggs, butter, red meat, whole milk, etc. and the food companies obliged by developing cholesterol-free products such as Egg Beaters ®, margarine, and other fat-free dairy products. Television advertising drove home the message that cholesterol was a killer substance, and any food product that was labeled "no cholesterol" was considered to be a life-saving substance. The subliminal effect of years of persistent advertising and the acquiescence of the overwhelming majority of physicians changed the eating habits of many millions of Americans.

For many years, the avante garde health enthusiasts who are variously called "faddists", "health food nuts or freaks", or just simply "quacks", have religiously maintained that good nutrition prevented disease. Academics and practicing physicians refuted those claims with the aforementioned epithets as they went about their business curing diseases with new drugs. It developed into a controversy over the advantages of prevention of disease versus its cure. It is in the context of this debate that the adoption of the "Lipid Hypothesis" seems so anomalous. Why has the medical establishment which has been so steadfast in its opposition to diet as a preventive measure in the etiology of disease suddenly seized upon an unproved theory, and with the ulterior motivation of the food industry succeeded in changing the dietary habits of our people? Can it be that the establishment has finally gotten religion? Is it possible that doctors now really believe that good nutrition can prevent disease? Have they joined hands with the quacks and advocate dietary improvement as a means of preventing disease?

The jury is still out on the cause of artery disease (atherosclerosis). We don't know the cause of heart disease. Heart attacks still persist as America's number one killer, and a low-cholesterol, low-fat diet is not a guarantee that you can avoid an attack. Cholesterol is a vital substance that is necessary for life itself. The liver normally produces about three times as much cholesterol as we get in our daily diet. To complicate the debate further, there are those who believe that the low-fat, low-cholesterol diet is ironically causing the disease that it is designed to prevent because it is denying us the good nutrition which we need to keep us in the best of health.

What Is Cholesterol?

To the average person, cholesterol is something that is bad and should be avoided at all costs. It is universally feared by the masses and it has unleashed a multi-billion dollar change in our food industry. The food architects have completely restructured the products that we eat today so that we can avoid the dreaded substance that will surely result in our early demise. Our diets have been altered with the insistence of our doctors to exclude any trace of cholesterol. These are the same people who never believed that nutrition had anything to do with disease. They now believe that avoiding cholesterol will somehow prevent heart disease.

It is true however, that the medical profession conceded that there were four cases where a deficiency of a vitamin or mineral caused a specific disease. Scurvy was caused by a lack of vitamin C, Beri-Beri by a deficiency of B-1 or Thiamine, Pellagra by a deficiency of B-3 or Niacin, and Rickets by a deficiency of vitamin D. It is difficult to expect anyone who isn't schooled in nutrition to champion its advocacy. Most doctors are trained to treat the symptom of a disease with a particular drug. They are loathe to admit that a vitamin can exert any influence on a patient's health and well-being. If you ask your doctor if it is all right to take vitamin and mineral supplements, he will invariable say, "It won't hurt you, but I personally think you are wasting your money. The truth is that you are flushing your money down the toilet!"

With that attitude about nutritional supplements and the almost nutrition-free diet that physicians prescribe to rid our blood of cholesterol, is it any wonder that we are experiencing an epidemic of degenerative diseases unprecedented in our history. If our immune system is deprived of the life-sustaining nourishment that it so sorely needs to fight off disease we are witnessing a double-whammy. Our doctors offer us a diet stripped of the nutrition we so desperately need and they tell us we don't need to supplement it with life-sustaining nutrients!

Now what is this cholesterol that we are told to avoid? It is a solid alcohol, a fat-like substance that is found in every living cell in the body. It is especially found in the brain. Two thirds of the dry weight of the brain is composed of cholesterol. The liver produces about 80 percent of the cholesterol we need for life. We get the rest from our diet. The liver regulates the cholesterol level. When more is consumed in the diet, less is manufactured by the liver.

Cholesterol is carried in the blood, which is a watery medium, yet it is not soluble in water. It is therefore combined with proteins and fats into giant molecules called "lipoproteins" which are water soluble. That is how cholesterol is carried in the blood. Cholesterol is therefore important because it plays a necessary role of transporting fats in the body. In fact, the liver makes cholesterol to match the amount of fat to be converted into lipoproteins and disposes of excess cholesterol by excreting it in the bile.

The Diet Dilemma

The relationship between diet and disease might have come to the fore over a century ago had not medical science become so elated with Pasteur's dramatic discovery that microbes cause disease. It took many painful years of effort and discovery for Pasteur to prevail. Although Pasteur never said that all diseases were caused by bacteria, many in the medical profession soon came to make that assumption.

When Eijkman, a Dutch physician, discovered that Beriberi was due to a nutritional deficiency, his discovery was rejected, leading him to discount his own conclusions in spite of his experiments. As late as 1898, Eijkman said that infection was the probable cause of disease, but during the next eight years, he changed his mind. Thirty-one years later, he received a Nobel Prize for the discovery of vitamin B-1. In 1911, Casimir Funk claimed that not only Beriberi, but Rickets, Scurvy, and Pellagra were caused by an unknown nutritional deficiency.

Diet is of the utmost importance to your health. Because medical education excludes cellular nutrition, physicians have not developed expertise in this area. Doctors are humane and dedicated, but they are also businessmen and women. If their patients stay healthy, physicians suffer financial loss. If doctors were paid only when we were well and we withheld payment when sick, the prevention of disease would flourish. The current situation is exacerbated by the fact that the pharmaceutical industry makes enormous profits from the sale of drugs; the drug companies are understandably not overly anxious to prevent diseases that would put them out of business. Yet the nutritional approach to medicine is valuable and necessary, and today's medical students must begin to change the entrenched attitudes and think more of health instead of concentrating on disease.

Many authorities attribute heart disease and the buildup

of plaque inside artery walls to cholesterol. At first glance, it would seem like a good idea to consume less cholesterol, but it is actually a very poor one. If we eliminate cholesterol, we sacrifice good nutrition and may thus be courting heart disease. Research reveals that good nutrition prevents cholesterol deposits from forming. It is important to remember that cholesterol is made within our bodies and can be deposited in our arteries even if no cholesterol is consumed at all.

Every food we eat should contribute in a positive way to develop a better nutritional environment. But what is most needed is an informed public that will raise its voice. Nutrients are a fundamental part of the chain of life; when the diet becomes deficient in nutrients, the chain is broken and the pathways are open to disease, premature aging, and unnecessary death.

Greed

In the 1920's, a Wall Street trader named Barnie Winkleman said, "Greed is stronger than sex." The power of money surely played an important role in the development and growth of the diet-cholesterol-coronary heart disease paradigm. While the early researchers were well-intentioned and seekers of truth, the decades that followed added many profit-driven industries to the lucrative "cholesterol business."

The American Heart Association is a nationwide, publicly funded organization. In the early 1950's, it ordered a study of the whole diet-cholesterol-CHD question. In 1957, the results of the study were disclosed. It revealed that there was overwhelming evidence that diet had no effect on blood (serum) cholesterol levels. What did the American Heart Association do? Nothing...for four years. It sat on the report and waited. Is it too much for the public which funds the studies the AHA does to expect the organization to demonstrate its honesty and integrity? The AHA had two choices. It could reveal the truth about the results of the study or it could do additional studies to confirm or reject the results. It did neither.

In 1961, the American Heart Association jumped on the diet-cholesterol-CHD bandwagon. This stand completely disregarded the study which had just been completed. The new diet recommendation was for a low-fat, low-cholesterol regimen which allowed only 3 eggs a week. This diet ostensibly would lead to a lower cholesterol level and prevent the development of CHD. Not only did the AHA know better, but it was playing with the lives of millions of Americans who are urged to avoid the most nutritious foods such as eggs, whole milk, beef, butter among others.

Thirty-five years and billions of dollars of research after the abandonment of integrity, the AHA continues to hew to the diet-cholesterol-CHD line. It ignores the vast accumulation of studies which betray the diet theory. Indeed, the mother of all heart studies which is now 49 years old, "The Framingham Heart Study", which is funded by the National Institutes of Health, has proved overwhelmingly that diet is not involved in the development of CHD.

In its 1970 study titled, "Diet and the Regulation of Serum Cholesterol", the Framingham researchers proclaim very clearly that dietary cholesterol does not increase blood (serum) cholesterol. They also stated that saturated fats did not increase blood cholesterol. It is troubling to see that these important findings, which are funded by public tax money have been carefully hidden from view for more than 25 years. Perhaps the researchers who commissioned the study were disappointed in the results. The findings did not confirm the consensus belief that diet could alter the inevitable rise in cholesterol that leads to CHD. Does science exist for the benefit of the researchers or is it meant to reveal the truth! The perpetuation of the diet-cholesterol-coronary heart disease paradigm can hardly give comfort to a confused public. It should be cause for consternation and wrath that tax monies are being squandered in ways that are self-serving, useless, and a danger to the health of our people.

The Homocysteine Revolution

The overwhelming resistance of the cholesterol/fat hierarchy is finally beginning to unravel. It took the dedication of a true scientist, who devoted his life to the search for the truth and the dissemination of the facts he discovered about the largest killer in the United States, coronary heart disease. His discovery is the central theme of a new book called, "The Homocysteine Revolution." Kilmer S. McCully M.D. discovered that an amino acid called Homocysteine is a strong independent risk factor for arteriosclerosis.

Homocystinuria is a disease that is characterized by hardening of the arteries. McCully studied the results of 10 cases in London and Belfast who had hardening of the arteries caused by Cystinuria. He was curious to know why there was no cholesterol deposited in the walls of the children's arteries? McCully hypothesized that an elevated homocysteine level caused the arteriosclerosis. This discovery was of tremendous importance because scientists in 1969 were searching for another approach to understanding coronary heart disease. There were many unanswered questions about the cholesterol paradigm. For example, why the majority of heart disease patients have a normal or low cholesterol?

McCully's ideas were denounced by the cholesterol camp. If accepted, it would undermine the conventional view of prevention and treatment of heart disease. But dietary cholesterol does not raise blood (serum) cholesterol. McCully knew that the Framingham Heart Study in 1970, showed that conclusion. He also knew that the children and animals with Homocystinuria had no cholesterol in their artery walls!

The vast majority of the medical community ignored the new homocysteine theory. It was not only radically different from the consensus but it would undermine the livelihood of the alliance that had developed over the decades including The American Heart Association, the governmental agencies such as The National Institutes of Health, The National Heart, Lung, and Blood Institute, the giant pharmaceutical industry, and the mammoth food industry. McCully was fighting a one trillion dollar colossus!

The Homocysteine approach is radically different from the cholesterol theory which believes that atherosclerosis develops from the dietary consumption of excessive amounts of fats and cholesterol. The homocysteine theory holds that arteries are damaged by the injurious effect of homocysteine on cells and tissues of the arteries, leading to loss of elasticity, hardening, calcification, narrowing of the lumen and formation of blood clots in the arteries. The homocysteine theory considers arteriosclerosis a disease of protein intoxication, the cholesterol theory considers the disease to be caused by intoxication from fats.

There is one major difference between the cholesterol paradigm and the homocysteine theory. McCully has discovered the means of preventing the buildup of blood homocysteine, thereby preventing arteriosclerosis. Prevention can be achieved by consumption of foods that provide an abundant supply of vitamin B-6, B-12 and Folic acid. Many factors contribute to the complex problem of coronary heart disease. Male gender, post menopause in women, genetics, smoking, sedentary life, high blood pressure and thyroid disease. There are many cases of severe arteriosclerosis in which cholesterol is normal. McCully believes that the major decline in the risk of stroke and heart attack since the mid 1960's could have been related to the increased vitamin B-6 in the food supply. Recent studies suggest that 50,000 American lives can be saved by adding Folic acid to the food supply.

For 80 years, the cholesterol/fat theory dominated the consensus. One of the major shortcomings of the cholesterol/

fat approach is the lack of an explanation for the rapid escalation of coronary heart disease and stroke during the mid-20th century in America and its dramatic decline in the mid 1960's. The American diet has changed very little during the recent decades which saw a two-to-three fold decline in coronary heart disease and stroke. Cholesterol levels were the same during this period.

The time lag in the medical world is always 50 to 100 years. There has to be "a paradigm shift" about the cause of arteriosclerosis. There are too many questions about the cholesterol theory which have no adequate answers. The success of the cholesterol-lowering statin drugs is compromised by evidence of liver and muscle toxicity and cancer in animals.*1 And evidence that these drugs inhibit the formation of ubiquinone, a key component of energy production in heart and other cells.*2

It was not until 1993 that a biochemical theory related the observations on homocysteine and vascular disease to observations in the cholesterol/fat field. Recent studies show widespread deficiencies of vitamin B-6, B-12 and Folic acid in elderly and cardiac patients. Rinehart's studies with monkeys showed very little fat and cholesterol in the arteriosclerotic plaques. They were fibrous and fibrocalcific.*4

The medical community refused to accept the homocysteine theory because it relegates cholesterol to a secondary role in the causation of coronary heart disease. The huge multi-billion dollar business that cholesterol has built is very lucrative and fraught with political intrigue. They won't give up easily. It will take an aroused public to stir their representatives into action.

The Hordaland Homocysteine Study concludes that we can view arteriosclerosis as a deficiency disease. The approach is revolutionary because for the last 50 years, artery disease was viewed as a disease of excess consumption of sugars, cholesterol and fats.*3 Folic acid will be added to foods in 1998 according to a decision of the United States Department of Agriculture. The dietary intake of vitamin B-12 is adequate for the population except for strict vegetarians. A future goal is to require the addition of B-6 to enrich foods which are lost in the processing. It will help continue the decline in arteriosclerosis and improve the general health and promote increased life expectancy in the population. Kilmer McCully says that the homocysteine blood level should be no higher than 14 micro moles. There is a blood test by Baxter Laboratories but it is not yet very accurate. There is no doubt that a new test will be developed as the public becomes aware of the homocysteine phenomenon.

*1 Thomas B. Newman and Stephen B. Hulley "Carcinogenicity of Lipid-lowering Drugs." JAMA 275:55-60 1996

*2 Willis Richard et al "Lovastatin Decrease Coenzyme Q10 Levels in Rats." Proceedings of the NAS USA 87: 8928-8930, 1990

*3 Ohar Nygard et al "Total Plasma Homocysteine and Cardiovascular Risk Profile." "The Hordaland Homocysteine Study" JAMA 274:1526-1533, 1995

*4 James F. Rinehart and Louis D. Greenberg, "Vitamin B-6 Deficiency in the Rhesus Monkey with Particular Reference to the Occurrence of Atherosclerosis, Dental Caries and Hepatic Cirrhosis." American Journal of Clinical Nutrition 4: 318-325, 1956.

Glucocide

The road to nutritional disaster began in the eighteenth century. That is the time when white bread came into general use. Refined sugar (sucrose) consumption started a dizzying climb from 15 pounds a year per person to a caloric sweetener total of 150 pounds per year in 1994. This represents a 1000 percent gain and almost 3 pounds a week for the average person. If you add the extra sugar consumed in the form of the starches like pasta, rice, and potatoes, the total swells to more than 200 pounds of sugar or about 4 pounds a week for the average person!

Dr. John Yudkin, the eminent British nutritionist, warned about the evils of sugar in his outstanding book, "Sweet and Dangerous." His research uncovered the danger of this massive consumption of refined white flour and table sugar. He claimed that sugar was responsible for atherosclerosis and coronary heart disease. His studies in a British hospital proved his theory was correct. He was disillusioned with the scientific community which never accepted his findings, and he recently passed away without ever receiving the credit he so richly deserved for his research.

The landmark work on the devastating effects of white flour and sugar is Surgeon-Captain T.L. Cleave's, "The Saccharine Disease." He claims that a master disease has evolved which is the cause of obesity, diabetes, coronary thrombosis, cancer of the colon, and other degenerative diseases. When steel rollers were introduced around the year 1880, a whiter flour was produced, and that period marked the emergence of Cleave's "Saccharine Disease."

Dr. Robert C. Atkins rails against the consumption of refined sugar and white flour on his radio programs, and one night he said, "Sugar is death!" Dr. Abram Hoffer, the Canadian Orthomolecular Psychiatrist, said in his book, "Nutrients to Age Without Senility," "The maximum amount of sugar an individual should eat is zero." Richard Passwater, Ph.D., in his book, "Supernutrition" calls sugar, "The Sweet Killer." The picture is clear, but not too much fuss is made about sugar in the media. The fear of cholesterol is a more appealing story for the public, and it sells food, drugs, and other products. It would be earth-shattering for the public to learn that sugar consumption to a great degree is responsible for increasing cholesterol levels.

Every spoonful of refined sugar you eat compromises your body's health, robbing you of the nutrients you need for metabolism and digestion. The minerals needed to digest sugar are chromium, manganese, cobalt, copper, zinc, and magnesium. They are stripped away in the refining process and the body has to deplete its own mineral reserves to use refined sugar. It is therefore an anti-nutrient.

Glucose is used as a cheap filler by the food industry in foods such as cereals, baked goods, sauces, and processed meats. It is an excellent preservative adding an extra benefit to the food processors. And there is no law requiring glucose to be listed as an ingredient on the label of any package, so even if you don't consume large amounts of sugar directly, you can experience problems. Hypoglycemia (low-blood sugar, arthritis, tooth decay, endocrine problems, diabetes, cancer, and all the degenerative diseases can be the result of a blood sugar imbalance.

A 10-ounce glass of orange juice has the equivalent of 9 teaspoons of sugar, the same as a 12-ounce can of coke. The soft drink industry has grown to a $62 billion dollar industry. The food industry does not support research on the effect of sugar on the body, since it relies on sugar for the manufacture of processed foods. The pharmaceutical industry, too, would only harm itself with research; if people stopped eating sugar they wouldn't need so many drugs.

Glucocide is a national terror. It is sweeping the country while it spreads its degenerative horror. We are literally eating our way to oblivion. Oceans of cola drinks, mountains of ice cream, hundreds of billions of dollars of cakes, cookies, pies, pretzels, potato chips, muffins, and doughnuts-the list is endless. The supermarket is leading us down the road to nutritional Armageddon—Glucocide—The White Death.

The Polyunsaturated Peril

The greatest myth behind the cholesterol controversy is the theory that if you eat polyunsaturated fats and cut out saturated fats your risk of having heart disease is reduced. There is no proof that this is so. The publicity campaign that has altered the American diet stresses polyunsaturated fats at the expense of meat, dairy products, and eggs.

The danger that develops when polyunsaturates are used in cooking they break down into free-radical compounds that combine with oxygen to form peroxides, which are really toxic substances. They damage the cells, their components, and other body proteins. The more polyunsaturates there are in the tissues, the more destruction occurs of healthy, active cells. This results in premature aging and its accompanying diseases.

Many Americans have radically changed their eating habits as a result of the overwhelming pressure of publicity from the American Heart Association and the advertising by corporations who profit from the sale of their products. The average person has increased his consumption of polyunsaturates more than 500% since 1920 (from 10 pounds to more than 50 pounds a year). While this was happening, the intake of animal fats (saturates) dropped from 20 pounds down to 10 pounds per person. All the while the cheerleaders of government agencies, food companies, and the American Heart Association encouraged this drastic dietary change on the country without knowing the disastrous consequences that would ensue.

The reaction of governmental agencies to the irresponsible and misleading advertising of polyunsaturated products is quite interesting. Although the FDA (Food and Drug Administration) is charged with the protection of the consumer from fraudulent health claims, it effectively passes this duty along to the FTC (Federal Trade Commission), which oversees advertising. The AMA (American Medical Association) decries the promotion of polyunsaturates as a health cure, yet its publications accept large sums of money for advertising claims that have no basis in fact.

The Federation of American Societies for Experimental Biology met in 1974 and Dr. Fred A. Kummerow and his colleagues from the University of Illinois at Urbana reported their studies on margarine. Newspapers carried the story under the title, "Margarine Found Health Hazard." The findings showed that a fat in margarine may present a greater health risk than cholesterol-rich foods such as beef fat, butterfat, and powdered eggs.

The researchers concluded that a hydrogenated fat which contains margarine base stock to make the product more stable (trans-fatty acids) was more atherogenic than the cholesterol-bearing foods mentioned above. The degree of atherosclerosis was determined by autopsies on experimental animals. Swine were used in the tests because the aorta and heart of a pig weigh about the same as those of a human, and pigs are close to humans in their response to cholesterol. The tests were repeated several times with identical results. The greatest degree of hardening of the arteries was in pigs fed margarine-base stock with their diet. The group fed sugar with their diet was next. The group fed butter had almost negligible damage, and the least disease was found in the groups fed egg yolks or egg whites with their standard diet.

It has been shown *1 that corn oil, rich in polyunsaturated triglyceride fatty acids, is carcinogenic. If this is the case, it would be impossible to reduce the carcinogenicity of polyunsaturated fats.

The potentially carcinogenic lipid peroxides are easily formed from polyunsaturated fats by auto-oxidation. Not only are they extremely toxic, but they also bind strongly to gastric mucosal cells.*2 It would seem reasonable, therefore, that there should be a standard for the content of lipid peroxides in fats. In establishing such a standard, care must be taken to ensure that the methods used measure both the existing peroxide content of the fat and the peroxide-forming capacity of the fat. The latter is reduced if a suitable permitted antioxidant is added. Vitamin E is the natural antioxidant which can be used to limit oxidation.

These toxic and potentially carcinogenic substances can be produced by heating polyunsaturated fats.*3 Benzpyrene has been detected in margarine and other fats but not in butter.*4

Not only is it important to supplement a diet high in polyunsaturated fats (corn oil), soybean oil etc.) With vitamin E, but it is important to increase the consumption of Biotin and vitamin B-12. This has become increasingly important with the meteoric rise of polyunsaturated fat consumption to an all-time record level of 50.5 pounds per person annually as of 1994.*5

Since many polyunsaturated fat-rich vegetable oils have a low content of vitamin A, it is important that food preparations based on these products are supplemented with vitamin A. Thus, the restriction on the addition of carotene to cooking margarines (which are used for table purposes by many people) should be lifted. It is realized that these particular margarines contain very little polyunsaturated fats.

"The Cholesterol Controversy" by the late Dr. Edward R. Pinckney and Cathey Pinckney points out the dangers of a high intake of polyunsaturated food products. A few of these dangers are listed below:

1. Some doctors have shown that polyunsaturates can cause more heart and artery disease than they prevent.
2. Dr. Denham Harman, Professor of Medicine and Biochemistry at the University of Nebraska College of Medicine, reports that unsaturated fats increase the possibility of atherosclerosis, cancer, and other diseases. Animals who eat more polyunsaturates die

sooner. Man's life-span can be shortened by 15 years with concentrated use of polyunsaturates.

3. The Research Foundation for Plastic Surgery in Los Angeles studied 1000 patients for more than 2 years. Of those whose diet was 10% polyunsaturates, 78% showed marked signs of premature aging of the skin and face; some looked 20 years older than their actual age.

4. Studies with animals given polyunsaturates (not in large amounts) have shown shortening of life span, premature aging, and development of high blood pressure. Another disease that developed was Amyloidosis, a condition characterized by a gelatin-like material being deposited in various parts of the body. Amyloidosis is believed to cause senility, arthritis, and other chronic conditions.

5. The Mayo Clinic found that patients who have breast cancer also have an increased amount of polyunsaturated fatty acids in their breast tissue and blood plasma.

6. It is generally agreed by scientists everywhere that any increase in polyunsaturates requires an increased amount of vitamin E.

7. Dr. David Kritchevsky of the Wistar Institute in Philadelphia, Pennsylvania has shown that when corn oil is heated for more than 15 minutes, it can contribute to the development of atherosclerosis. Yet no one warns the public not to cook with these oils.

8. Dr. Neil R. Artman of the Procter & Gamble company admitted that polyunsaturated fats can be made nutritionally undesirable by heating and oxidation. Heating forms peroxides, which are toxic. This report was delivered to the American Heart Association in November 1970, but for some unknown reason was never released to the public or the medical profession.

The preponderance of evidence which indicts partially hydrogenated vegetable fats in the development of cancer should be enough to invoke the Delaney Clause of the American Food and Drug Law. The law states that material that causes cancer in any animal in any dose must not be used in any food. With more than 6 billion pounds of shortenings and cooking oil consumed every year, and the bulk of the fast food restaurants frying chicken, fish, potatoes etc., a frightening prospect confronts the American public. The domination of commercial interests is unfortunately causing a serious health hazard to an unaware public. Cancer rates are increasing as the consumption of polyunsaturates mount in a seemingly never-ending spiral. As noted before, vegetable fat consumption has grown from 10 pounds per person in 1920 to 50.5 pounds per person in 1990. This is an increase of more than 500 %.

The facts are staring us in the face. The lessons are clear. The proof is incontrovertible. What will it take for our leaders to take the bull by the horns and change our march toward nutritional disaster. When will truth overtake the greed that puts the public at risk for heart disease and cancer? One can only hope that the medical community will come to its senses and pay heed to the Hippocratic Oath to which all physicians pledge, "First-Do No Harm."

*1 Szepsenwol Proc. Amer Assoc. Cancer Research 12-94 (1971)

*2 Bergan, J.C. and Draper, H.H. Lipids 5,976 (1970)

*3 Michael, W.R., Alexander, J.C. and Artman, N.R. Lipids 1, 353 (1966)

*4 Fabian, B. Arch. Hyg. Bakt. 152, 231 (1968)

*5 Kummerow, F.A., Ph.D. "Viewpoint On The Report of the NCEP Expert Panel on Detection, Evaluation, and Treatment of High Blood Cholesterol in Adults" Journal of the American College of Nutrition Vol. 12, No. 1, 2-13 (1993)

Cholesterol or Nothing

The following is an analytical review of an article which appeared in Healthmap Magazine on December 1994. It was written by Dr. Robert C. Atkins, Founder and Director of the Atkins' Center in New York.

The National Cholesterol Education program (NCEP) which is funded by the National Institutes of Health continues to propagate the mainstream recommendation that lowering cholesterol will reduce the risk of heart disease. Dr. Atkins' maintains that following this advice would expose his patients to unnecessary risks from unsafe pharmaceuticals and subject himself to ridicule from those complementary physicians who know better.

The NCEP fails to realize that the diet it is recommending contains a good deal of carbohydrate consumption which increases the Triglyceride levels and is therefore a heart disease risk. This lack of the fundamental knowledge of nutrition makes the dietary advice of the authors suspect.

There have been six major studies since 1968 using diet and drugs to show that reducing cholesterol saves lives. In total nearly 25,000 men were tested. Only two studies included women. During the cholesterol-lowering period, there were 28 fewer deaths from coronary heart disease (169 compared to 197). This was more than offset by 36 more deaths from cancer and 29 violent deaths. This an excess of 33 deaths in the treated group.

The favorite drug in the cholesterol industry is Lovastatin or Mevacor. A study with Lovastatin involving 8,245 people at 362 hospital centers. 36 people died during this one-year study, almost all of them from heart disease. Only three of the people who died were not receiving Lovastatin. That means the people receiving drug therapy for high cholesterol had a 267% increase over those who were not treated. Heart attacks were fatal to 60 percent of the people in the drug therapy group compared to only one out of six in the group not receiving any kind of therapy. In another drug study, the results were even worse. A drug called Clofibrate was used in a study and the subjects were watched for 10 years after the drug treatment. The death from heart attacks among the men increased dramatically. 34 of them died of heart disease compared to 14 in the untreated group.

The NCEP is way behind the curve because new research is looking at three of the real culprits in heart disease. They are oxidized LDL cholesterol, homocysteine, and syndrome X. The oxidation of cholesterol can be reversed with the supplementation of vitamin E, Beta-carotene, Vitamin C, Selenium, and Coenzyme Q10. Homocysteine is considered a more accurate and reliable gauge of heart attacks than high cholesterol according to a study published in the New England Journal of Medicine 1991; 324: 149-155. All one has to do is to take B-6, Betaine, and Folic acid and you can achieve a tenfold greater reduction in heart disease risk than the NCEP program. Dr. Gerald Reaven's research at Stanford University (Diabetes, 1988; 37:1595-1607), demonstrates that resistance to the effect of insulin involves high blood levels of insulin, blood sugar irregularities, high triglycerides, high blood pressure, and obesity. Each of these conditions increases the risk of heart disease. It is obvious that the low-fat, low-cholesterol regimen recommended by the NCEP makes syndrome X worse.

How can the NCEP recommend a pat of margarine seven times a day? Does the panel know that the trans-fatty acids (partially hydrogenated vegetable oil) has been implicated in the development of heart disease? Dozens of studies (including Circulation, 1994: 89: 94-101) have shown this effect. The most well-known, the Harvard Nurses Study of 85,000 people found that people who eat margarine have a 66% greater chance of heart disease than those who don't eat the substance.

The NCEP could not complete its program without a warning about eggs. The panel suggests no-yolk egg-white omelets. This will help you miss out completely on the heart benefits of phospholipids which help the body's biological membrane function, and increase HDL.

The NCEP eliminates from its analysis the most significant studies in which 16,000 people participated. The Helsinki Study (Journal of the American Medical Association, 1991; 286: 1225-1229) which followed up subjects for 15 years showed that the death rate from heart disease among the people using drugs exceeded the death rate among the drugless group by 242 percent. This proves the NCEP's blind acceptance of the pharmaceutical treatment regardless of the actual results on human beings. Despite Atkins' warnings about drugs, he asks you to discuss these studies with your doctor and ask him or her to wean you off the prescription drugs. As nutrients nourish your heart and triglycerides decrease, and HDL increases, your physician will see that cholesterol medication can be reduced or eliminated.

Scientists Ease Up on Fear of Eggs
by Gina Kolata

When it comes to eggs, few medical experts are neutral. Either they want to see the entire population, young, old, women, children, those with low cholesterol levels, assiduously restricting egg consumption. Or they dismiss the anti-egg movement as so much dogmatism by heart disease fanatics.

The trusth, as scientists now view it seems to be not in the middle but more to the side of those who would like to see Americans relax about eggs—a sentiment that is growing.

Yes, eggs contain about 215 milligrams of cholesterol in their yolks.

Yes, cholesterol in the diet is capable of raising the levels of cholesterol in the blood.

But individual responses to cholesterol in food vary so greatly that some people show virtually no effect. And in any event, the primary culprit is not cholesterol in the diet but saturated fat in the diet: eating foods like red meat, which are high in saturated fat, has been shown to affect cholesterol levels in the blood powerfully. Eating eggs, which are hight in cholesterol, concerns many nutritional experts far less.

It turns out that the body makes its own cholesterol, which is an essential component of cell membranes and a key ingredient in hormone manufacture. So there is a balancing act. The more cholesterol you eat, the less your body makes. It's not a perfect balane: for some people the cholesterol level will rise if they eat more, said Dr. Ronald M. Krauss, the head of the department of molecular and nuclear medicine at the Donner Laboratory at the University of California, Berkeley.

But two studies by Dr. Henry N. Ginsberg at Columbia University's College of Physicians and Surgeons found that young men and women who ate as many as three to four eggs a day for weeks on end had virtually no change in their blook cholesterol levels.

The case against saturated fat, however, is strong. It decreases the body's ability to break down the cholesterol it takes in and can increase the rate at which the body synthesizes cholesterol, noted Dr. Alice H. Lichtenstein, a nutrition researcher at Tufts University. "The major determinant of plasma cholesterol levels is saturated fat," she said.

So who should worry about how many eggs they eat? Dr. Scott Grundy, director of the Center for Human Nutrition at the University of Texas, Southwestern School of Medicine in Dallas, is one of those who say that even those at low risk of heart disease should eat, on average, no more than three or four eggs yolks a week. It is prudent to develop eating habits that will help keep your cholesterol in check, he said.

Others, like Dr. David Kritchevsky, nutritional biochemist at the Wistar Institute in Philadelphia, maintain that the hazards of eggs are greatly exaggerated.

"Eggs are good for you," he said, and he eats as many as he pleases—many one week, few the next, unconcerned about egg cholesterol. "I don't think about it ever." Dr. Krauss, who is also the chairman of the American Heart Association's nutrition board said that most of the population—children, people with low cholesterol levels, women younger than 50 and men younger than 40—should not let fear of the almighty egg rule their lives. "I think there are more important things to worry about," he said.

Even for those who are at high risk of heart disease, Dr. Krauss puts eggs low on the list of worries. "In terms of diet, the biggest concern remains saturated fat and, more important, obesity," he said.

Why is Animal Fat Bad For Human Beings?
By Warren M. Levin, M.D., FAAFP, FACN, FAAEM

The good fat/bad fat controversy is inextricably bound up with the cholesterol theory of coronary artery disease. That's because there is really good "scientific" statistical evidence of a correlation between the high intakes of animal fats—which are high in cholesterol—with coronary artery disease (and other manifestations of hardening of the arteries), cancer of the colon, cancer of the prostate, and cancer of the breast. However, the composition of animal fat in terms of the fatty acids and cholesterol that it is made of hasn't changed for hundreds of thousands of years. Nevertheless, the incidence of all of the diseases enumerated above has skyrocketed just in the last half of this century! Another interesting statistic is that the number of heart attacks is remarkably correlated to the number of radios in this country! I would like to speak for a small but growing group of scientists who believe that it isn't the fat that God put in animals from time immemorial that is the cause of the problems (including cholesterol), but rather the contamination of that pristine healthy animal fat with man-made chemicals. In the last fifty years, since Upton Sinclair's powerful expose of the meat markets in Chicago (The Jungle), things have gotten steadily worse for the animals and the humans that eat them. Today, the intention of the cattle raising barons is to make the beef fatter faster. By experimentation they have discovered changes from the ancestral diet that encourage this deposition of "marbling" which makes the meat succulent and therefore more flavorful, and therefore more capable of fetching a higher price per pound—even though the protein content is relatively less than that of leaner animals. In addition to this drastic change in the content of the diet, the animals are housed so that they are unable to move around, making them bovine couch potatoes, so that they burn up less calories, and therefore accumulate even more weight as fat. The food that is supplied to these sedentary animals comes from farms whose goal is to produce maximum yield per acre. The agricultural scientists have created a mega industry in providing animal feed to the cattle raising industry. The agricultural scientist discovered in this century that artificial fertilizers stimulate the more rapid growth of plants to a larger size than the "old fashioned natural fertilizers." Unfortunately, these aberrations of the plant kingdom provide less nutrients and also tend to be more susceptible to their natural enemies, the various kinds of insects. That created another mega industry—pesticides. Naturally, the crops, once harvested were also more susceptible to the various and sundry molds and smuts, typical of stored grains. Ergo, the fungicide industry. The animals eating substandard food, unable to exercise, became susceptible to infectious diseases—it was a wonderful coincidence then that the antibiotics that were required to control infections seemed to also increase the fat content of the animals! And, just to enhance the growth rate even further, various hormones are fed to these hapless creatures.

And so, the stage is set for the final insult that I believe is the underlying cause of the statistical aberration that has unfairly laid the blame for cancer on animal fat: All of the aforementioned interventions are fat soluble chemicals, and they therefore concentrate in the fatty tissue of these animals. Most of these artificial substances behave in the body like weak estrogens! They are not, however, the natural estrogen that is healthful for the body—these artificial unnatural estrogens are probably the trigger—the cause—of the increased incidence of cancer. Every healthy man and woman that has ever walked the earth has had natural human estrogens circulating in the blood stream and bathing all of the cells. The highest levels occur in pregnant women. Nature doesn't cause pregnant women to carry high levels of a cancer

causeing hormone during pregnancy! The animals themselves don't live long enough to develp cancer—they are
raised for slaughter. It is the next step on the food chain—we
human beings—that further concentrate these toxins in our
system and express the increased propensity to develop
cancer. The chemicals also trigger Free Radical production
and thus contribute to coronary artery disease.

And what about the cholesterol in animal fat? It is a
necessary factor for both the animals and mankind. It plays a
critically essential role in the cell membranes of all of the
cells in animal bodies. Its time we stopped blaming nature for
causing cancer and heart disease with animal fat—Mother
Nature and Father God didn't make such a stupid mistake!

The bottom line: Eat organic meat, fowl, and eggs—as
Nature intended!

For Reference: "Our Stolen Future: Are We Threatening
Our Fertility, Intelligence and Survival" Theo Colborn -
World Wildlife Fund, 1996.

Warren M. Levin, MD, FAAFP, FACN, FAAEM

Bibliography

1. The Cholesterol Myth - Thomas J. Moore
   The Atlantic Monthly September 1989
2. The Cholesterol Controversy - Edward R. Pinckney, M.D. and Cathey Pinckney Sherbourne Press 1974
3. Nutrients to Age Without Senility - Abram Hoffer M.D., Ph.D. and Morton Walker   D.P.M. Keats Publishing Inc. 1980
4. The Cholesterol Conspiracy - Russell L. Smith Ph.D. Warren H. Green Inc. 1993
5. Mental and Elemental Nutrients - Carl C. Pfeiffer M.D., Ph.D.
   Keats Publishing Inc. 1975
6. The Best of Health Sheldon Zerden
   Four Walls Eight Windows 1989
7. How to Live Longer and Feel Better Linus Pauling W.H. Freeman and Company 1986
8. Lick the Sugar Habit Nancy Appleton Ph.D. Avery Publishing Group Inc. 1988
9. Dr. Atkins' Health Revolution Robert C. Atkins M.D. Houghton Mifflin Company 1988
10. The Saccharine Disease Surgeon-Captain T.L. Cleave Keats Publishing Inc. 1976
11. Food For Naught: The Decline in Nutrition - Ross Hume Hall Vintage Books
12. Supernutrition for Healthy Hearts - Richard Passwater Ph.D. The Dial Press
13. Solved: The Riddle of Illness - Stephen E. Langer M.D. With James F. Scheer Keats Publishing Inc. 1984
14. Nutrition Against Disease Roger J. Williams Ph.D. Bantam Books 1973
15. Controlling Cholesterol Kenneth H. Cooper M.D., M.P.H. Bantam Books 1988
16. The Living Heart Diet - Michael DeBakey M.D.,

Antonio M. Gotto Jr., Lynne W. Scott, and John P. Foreyt

17. The Exercise Myth   Henry A. Solomon M.D. Harcourt Brace Jovanovich 1984

18. Coronary Heart Disease: The Dietary Sense and Nonsense-An Evaluation by Scientists-Edited by George V. Mann Sc.D., M.D.,-For the Veritas Society 1991

19. Sweet and Dangerous John Yudkin, M.D. Bantam Books 1973

20. The Cholesterol Humbug   Jerome Gillman The National Commission on Egg Nutrition 1978

21. Cholesterol & Your Health: The Great American Rip Off Chris Mudd American Lite 1990

22. Dr. Atkins' New Diet Revolution Robert C. Atkins M.D. M. Evans & Company 1992

23. The Homocysteine Revolution, Kilmer S. McCully, M.D.; Keats Publishing, Inc., 1997

FOR OTHER
TITLES
CALL
800-729-4131